The Me You Don't Know

A Gift of Knowledge for My Future Caregivers

Providing future caregivers the most important facts about your life

Dee Marrella

DC PRESS
A Division of the Diogenes Consortium
SANFORD • FLORIDA

Published by DC Press, 2445 River Tree Circle, Sanford, FL 32771
http://www.focusonethics.com

For general information on our other products and services please contact our offices at 407-688-1156 and/or go to www.focusonethics.com.

Dee Marrella authored *Who Cares: A Loving Guide for My Future Caregivers*. That book has been replaced by this new publication. It utilizes the best of *Who Cares* and adds additional features that expand on the original book and provides a wider coverage of the topic.

This book was set in Adobe Goudy Old Style
Cover Design and Composition by Jonathan Pennell

Library of Congress Catalog Number: 2008937091
Marrella. Dee,
The Me You Don't Know: A Gift of Knowledge for Future Caregivers
ISBN: 978-1-932021-36-3

First DC Press Edition
Printed in the United States of America
10 9 8 7 6 5 4 3 2

This book is lovingly dedicated
to my mother, Beatrice Delia —
A happy person who suffered so much in her later years.

To my sisters,
Terry Nicoletti and Karen Wiesen —
Together, we tried our very best.

To my daughters, Tammy Toso,
Lani Martin and Robin Russo —
Your love and support during a very
trying time will never be forgotten.

To the love of my life, Len —
You encouraged me to care for my Mom.
You shared my stress and pain.
For this I am forever grateful.

To all who have shared your experiences with me.
You give me the inspiration to keep spreading the message
of loving care.

To future caregivers — May this book
help make the journey less stressful.

REGARDING
WHO CARES: A LOVING GUIDE FOR MY FUTURE CAREGIVERS

DEE MARRELLA was the author of the highly popular book *Who Cares: A Loving Guide for My Future Caregivers*. That book was reprinted many times and got into the hands of thousands upon thousands of people throughout North America. The publisher wanted all readers/users of this new book to understand why the transition was made from the original book to this new one. It is very important for everyone to understand our motivation.

The Me You Don't Know: A Gift of Knowledge for My Future Caregivers is the offspring, if you will, of the original title. It grew out of the success of *Who Cares* and also the need to expand the coverage and span a wider audience of readers/users. The vast majority of people who acquired the first book were in the age group of 60+. Obviously younger people also put the book to use, but we saw a great need to reach readers in their mid- to late twenties through the mid-fifties. Our experience taught us that the material presented and the scope of the book would and should serve audiences ranging from the mid-twenties through post-retirement.

And so we created a new book — one that took the best of *Who Cares* and added new material to fit that wider audience base and to provide future caregivers with even more important information about and insight into YOU.

—DC Press

RED ALERT

VERY IMPORTANT

Note: Take a half dozen sheets of 8 1/2" x 11" blank paper and recreate the **RED ALERT** list found on the next two pages. Fill out the **RED ALERT** sheets completely, fold them and place them in the rear of this guide book so that the top of the sheet and the words **RED ALERT** can be easily seen. The words **RED ALERT** should be visible above the pages of the book and visible to anyone using the book for vital information concerning the person receiving attention. The information on this **RED ALERT** is ***critical*** information that you would want anyone who found you to have quick access.

Your RED ALERT should begin with the following:

"On this page I am listing ***Very Important*** information about myself. Please refer to it when any emergency situation arises."

IN CASE OF EMERGENCY

My Name: ____________________

My Social Security Number: ____________________

My birth date and current age: ____________________

My blood type: ____________________

Key Persons to Contact

Name: ____________________

Relationship: ____________________

Address: ____________________

Telephone # (Office): ____________________

Telephone # (Home): ____________________

Cell #: ____________________

Name: ____________________

Relationship: ____________________

Address: ____________________

Telephone # (Office): ____________________

Telephone # (Home): ____________________

Cell #: ____________________

Key Persons to Contact (Continued)

Name: ______________________________

Relationship: ______________________________

Address: ______________________________

Telephone # (Office): ______________________________

Telephone # (Home): ______________________________

Cell #: ______________________________

Name: ______________________________

Relationship: ______________________________

Address: ______________________________

Telephone # (Office): ______________________________

Telephone # (Home): ______________________________

Cell #: ______________________________

Name: ______________________________

Relationship: ______________________________

Address: ______________________________

Telephone # (Office): ______________________________

Telephone # (Home): ______________________________

Cell #: ______________________________

I am allergic to the following drugs:

I am allergic to the following foods:

I am being treated for: (fill in with illness, condition, disease, i.e, Diabetes):

LIST OF CURRENT MEDICATIONS/DOSAGE

Name: ______________________

Dosage: ______________________

Name: ______________________

Dosage: ______________________

Name: ______________________

Dosage: ______________________

Name: ______________________

Dosage: ______________________

Name: ______________________

Dosage: ______________________

Name: ______________________

Dosage: ______________________

Name: ______________________

Dosage: ______________________

Name: ______________________

Dosage: ______________________

My Personal Physician is:

Name: ______________________________

Hospital Affiliation: ______________________________

Telephone #: ______________________________

My Pharmacy is:

Name: ______________________________

Address: ______________________________

Telephone #: ______________________________

Durable Power of Attorney/Living Will:

Who has copy: ______________________________

Location: ______________________________

Telephone #: ______________________________

NOTE: Create these RED ALERT forms and have them ready for use at any time. Keep the most current version of this form folded with the RED ALERT facing out and inserted into the back of this guide or placed in a location that emergency responders can easily spot them. Keep this RED ALERT current. Consider using a pencil in areas that will change periodically.

ATTENTION

1. No matter what your age — complete this book NOW — not later. Don't put it away on a shelf until **completed**.
2. Place this guide where future caregivers can easily access vital information such as — where medications are specifically located.
3. Every individual being told by his/her doctor that they have the beginning stages of Alzheimer's or dementia should complete this book.
4. Military personnel being deployed anywhere in the world (hostile or not) should complete a copy. It may be difficult to imagine, but one can be seriously injured and find him or herself being taken care of for the remainder of his or her life.
5. Update the contents once a year, if possible. (Very few things will change.)
6. Remember to tell your caregivers that they are all just human beings. If they have done all they can to love you, comfort you, and help you maintain your dignity — they can not do more.
7. If you are a parent of a child with special needs, one of your concerns is "Who will take care of my child if I become seriously ill or die first?" By filling out a copy of this book for that child, in addition to completing one for yourself, you will have provided all future caregivers with valuable information about the habits, needs, and interests of the child — as well as providing some peace of mind for yourself.

CONTENTS

PART II: MY HEALTHCARE 25

PART III: PREFERENCES 51

PART IV: MY FINANCES 99

PART V: PERSONAL HISTORY 139

PREFACE

I WAS PRIVILEGED to be my mother's caregiver for five years. During that time, my Mother and I laughed and cried together. She did not want to be sick, and I didn't want her to be sick.. However, we agreed to deal with a difficult situation in the most positive manner possible.

I can honestly say that I am a better person today for having been a caregiver.

- First, I discovered patience I didn't know I possessed.
- An appreciation developed inside me for good people who came forward to help during those very difficult years.
- It became crystal clear that a sense of humor can transform a difficult situation into a tolerable one.

Humor is a way of fending off our own fears.

- I learned to have more tolerance and empathy of others.

When I look back, I realize those five years as my Mom's caregiver were the most emotionally filled years of my life. I felt as though I was in a bumper car at an amusement park — things were somewhat normal and suddenly I'd be hit from behind and forced to make a serious decision on the spot. Then things would be "OK" for a time, just before I'd be hit on the side and have to make another decision and try another path with her care. I was always tense and poised to react on my Mother's behalf. So many times I wished I could get her input on what she would have wanted. All I could do was guess. Dementia had taken over.

When you get the call that there has been an accident, illness or catastrophe, your life changes on the spot. You are now the president and CEO of another person's life and their well being. Caregiving is an awesome responsibility! That is why I wrote the first edition of this book back in 2002. I knew, from experience, what is involved in caregiving and I wanted to provide a hands-on guide – a roadmap – to help my daughters when (not "if") I ever needed their help. When they used the book, I wanted to be able to guide them and assist when they had to make those many decisions — large and small — that lay ahead. With book in hand, they could see my instructions — written in my own handwriting — and understand my very personal wishes and desires.

"What are my fears?" "What are my wishes regarding healthcare?" "How is my pet to be cared for?" "What is my favorite ice cream flavor?" "How do I feel about my doctors and other healthcare providers?"

These and many more questions about YOU will be answered when you fill out this book. When completed, your future caregivers will be able to live with less guilt and more peace of mind — and you will rest easier knowing that you still have a say in your own destiny.

WHO SHOULD COMPLETE THIS BOOK?

- **Young Parents**

  Remember 9/11? The majority of victims were under the age of retirement. Most of these victims left no will. They had never created directives for their loved ones. Illness or catastrophe were not words that most of them allowed to cross their minds. But as America discovered that day, catastrophe can strike when least expected. Planning ahead prevents confusion and many regrets. All it takes is an auto accident, a stroke (which doesn't respect age or sex), or major illness to rock one's world. Certainly young parents don't have much time to consider these types of events. However, most would agree that auto insurance, house or renters insurance, health insurance, and life insurance are necessities and worth the expense – especially when they are put to use. If you agree, then understand the importance of putting your thoughts, wishes and desires down on paper for your spouse, significant other, parents, and children – so they won't find themselves arguing over what they thought you might want.

- **Individuals Diagnosed with Early Dementia or Alzheimer's**

  This is an invaluable tool for future caregivers, especially when that person can no longer speak for himself or herself. It can be comforting to know that the book they completed can speak for them when they no longer can.

Parents of Special Needs Children

So often one hears parents of children with special needs express concern that the children will outlive them. Who will care for those children after the parents are gone? What will the level of care be for them? Filling out the pages in this book "for the child" will provide some peace of mind for the parents —knowing that they've provided insight into who their child is and guidelines for caring for that individual in the future. While no single source can address all that goes through the mind of concerned parents, this book can serve as one link to give their child a better life in the future when the parents aren't around.

Aging Americans

Many illnesses that were once fatal are now chronic. Americans are living longer. And when illness, disease and disabilities are prolonged through various life extension methods, this means that more of us will require long-term care. Our future caregivers will need our guidance more than we can imagine. We need to be prepared. This book will constitute one of our many preparations.

Military Personnel

Our sons and daughters (perhaps YOU) are actively protecting our country on many fronts. Many soldiers return from foreign deployments with serious and life-threatening injuries and increasing numbers of veterans will require life-long care. But as we all know, one doesn't have to be in a war zone to be serious injured. That can happen in any friendly environment. Nevertheless, the need to be prepared can not be overstated. This book, filled out prior to any deployment, could help a future caregiver in so many valuable ways — if needed, when needed.

I wrote this book in hopes of providing my own future caregivers with a guide that will serve them well. I wanted them to be able to open the book, refer to specific pages, and know exactly what I would want in a given situation — thus allowing them to be *informed caregivers* instead of *confused interpreters*. I refer to this book as "Love Insurance."

It doesn't cost anything but time to fill out the pages. But I promise — upon completion, the benefits are spectacular.

NOTE: If you are comfortable discussing the completed book with your future caregivers (if you have the opportunity to know who they might be), it can open many doors for all types of discussions. Allow your future caregivers to become familiar with *The Me You Don't Know* and where it can be located in your home. Working together now will benefit all concerned later.

FOREWORD

OUR AMERICAN POPULATION IS AGING. This is well known and seems to be discussed everywhere with new medications and treatments to combat the illnesses and conditions that afflict us as we grow older. Debilitating conditions affecting the young are also on the rise including Multiple Sclerosis, Muscular Dystrophy, Parkinsonism, and Autism to name a few. As medical science continues to advance, new treatments are discovered for these conditions as well. While these advancements are wonderful, it can be confusing for our family and caregivers to remember over the years which treatments worked best for us, which ones did not, and which ones we are currently taking. It is vital to your life and to your quality of living that your family and caregivers have this information readily available, so they don't have to rely on their memory in times of stressful decisions, anguished guilt, and heart-wrenching grief.

This book, ***The Me You Don't Know***, ensures that they won't forget. It is a reference book about YOU. When completed, it contains all pertinent information about you in one convenient location: Your personal likes and dislikes, your personal beliefs, physical problems, medications and allergies, family medical history, favorite brand of personal products (such as toothpaste and soap), wishes for medical treatment and life support, preferred healthcare providers (such as doctor and dentist), daily routine, favorite foods, hobbies, clothing sizes and preferences, favorite forms of entertainment, and favorite places to visit. This is just a partial listing. The scope of information in this book is amazing.

In completing the book, ***The Me You Don't Know***, you can give to your family and caregivers the information they need about you—your medical history and medications, favorite foods and least favorite foods, suggestions for gifts you would like and places to visit. For parents of physically and developmentally challenged children, it is a communication tool for your child's next caregiver—family member, friend or hired professional—to ensure that they have the information they need to care for your child when you need a short break from their care or a more permanent arrangement.

Today, this book provides personal and practical information regarding your care or that of your child. In the future, it will provide for your descendents a window into the past to YOU. Your children, grandchildren, and possibly countless descendents will have the opportunity to know you—your lifestyle, your values, and even your pets.

This book is an encyclopedia about YOU—the YOU that perhaps no one else knows: life lessons you have learned, beliefs and moral values, and yes, your regrets. By including these areas Dee Marrella has created a guidebook that encompasses the whole person in addition to medical facts, making this a treasured practical document today and a family heirloom tomorrow.

—**Marian R. Kranz, PT**
Geriatric Physical Therapist, Bellevue, WA

Loving

Kindness

Compassion…

Begin with me

AUTHOR'S COMMENT

CAREGIVERS need guidelines on how to comfort and care for a loved one. When individuals become our caregivers, they should have ***our*** input available to them. We all worry about wills, funerals, and leaving finances in order — ***for after we die***. This book is focused on lessening pain and stress when we become ill or incapacitated.

This book is designed to be filled out by the individual for whom future care is intended. This book is a person's chance to direct not only the care they will receive, but the "who's, what's, when's where's and how's" of his or her daily life.

By filling this book out, you have more control over your own destiny. You will also have given a great gift to your loved ones — peace of mind.

Maybe it is not comfortable for you to discuss this with your caregivers. Maybe it is not comfortable for them either. Maybe you cannot even tell them you have prepared this book for their use. You can, however, leave it with important papers, on your desk, where you stash your unpaid bills, under your address book, where you keep your car keys or medication. In other words, you can leave it where they are bound to find it when suddenly there is a need to take care of you and handle your affairs. Either way, they will have it and be able to be guided by your wishes.

If you are one of the lucky individuals who can discuss your wishes with your future caregivers, this book can help open all kinds of doors. If possible give it to your future caregiver now. Ask them to become familiar with it. Invite them to ask you questions. Invite them to make notes in it. Remember: this is a living document in more ways than one.

The guide is divided into various sections. I have made every effort to anticipate all the categories that affect your life — not merely the big decisions, but all the little things that enhance the quality of each day.

Because this is a tool that I too have been using and filling out for my own children, there are places throughout the book where I have jumped right in and provided you, the reader, with sample answers. These are my answers for my children. They are there to give you an idea of the scope or detail you may wish to provide in your own responses to your future caregivers. Your responses will certainly be your own.

At the end, I have added an extra chapter. To supplement the specific guidlines you provide your caregivers, I offer some general guidance that can help all of our future caregivers.

After the final chapter, there is a section called "Notes." This contains a grouping of blank pages that I promised earlier. I am sure you will think of categories that I've not included, that apply to you and your own special needs and requests. You might simply need additional space to complete comments from an earlier chapter. Make these pages your own.

Another addition is one I call 'Words and Phrases To Keep Handy.' Here you will find some important terms with which you should be familiar.

There are two important reasons for an individual to fill this book out:

1. You can have some control over your future destiny
2. Your decendants will benefit. This book will record things that will help trace family genetic and medical history.

— **Dee Marrella**

You can reach Dee at ***dee@themeyoudontknow.com***.

PUBLISHER'S COMMENT

INDEPENDENT PUBLISHERS hope that they'll publish a book that so many people love that it goes into a second edition. It isn't often that the wish comes true. At the same time, you might imagine how very happy a publisher might be if that same book went into a third edition. That's what happened over the years with ***Who Cares***. We actually reprinted the first edition some fifteen times and the second edition another seven. It was that success and the obvious need to reach a broader audience that we created ***The Me You Don't Know***.

Over the years I've been proud to receive the snail mail, emails and phone calls that have come in from individuals, family members, and professionals (attorneys, accountants and physicians) who have shared wonderful stories of their experiences with the book or people they knew who had put the book to work — the way it was designed to work. This new edition contains revised, expanded, and new material that have been provided by some of those people. Knowing that our original concept — empowering people to become a proactive voice in their own future caregiving — has been embraced by thousands of people across this country (and in Canada) has given me a great feeling inside. However, without the original concept and drive of Dee Marrella, I don't know if the book would have ever come to life.

The Me You Don't Know is an ever-evolving project. I doubt that it will ever end. There will always be a tremendous need on the part of all of us to want to be heard when the day comes that we find ourselves in the hands of caregivers. Each new year provides new practices and procedures that impact healthcare and how individuals are cared for. With each new year, each of us has more information to deal with and more personal information to share. Without a prepared guide for those who will care for us — people we can't even imagine, our chances of "being heard" becomes slim. What we've provided in this new edition will stand solidly with each person who takes the time to complete the pages and tell those future unknown people "everything" about themselves.

As I stated in the first edition, youth gives most of us the false sense that life has no limits with no end in sight. Little time is spent contemplating old age or some future illness or disability. However, by the time mid-life hits us, most people find it all quite shocking. I've often told people that "I went to bed the other night and I was just 18. When I woke up, I wasn't." Time flies by and the years pile up. Before long, we are dealing with challenges we were never educated about and are unprepared to face.

So allow me to make it very clear: this book is for every adult — regardless of age. Age has nothing to do with the need to prepare for the future. Let me illustrate:

- We don't dream of taking our new car and smashing it into another vehicle at an intersection on a rainy afternoon. Nevertheless, we have auto insurance just for those situations

- Few people sit around considering when they will die — especially when they are just starting their lives, just got married, or starting a new career. Yet, the majority of American carry life insurance. And many make benefits associated with the jobs (such as health and life insurance) part of the reason they stick with a company.

- While none of us are eager to come down with a serious illness or anticipate living with a disability, health insurance surely plays a significant part in our everyday lives.

- And when the biggest purchase of our lives occurs — buying a house, we insure it against all manner of potential perils. But we surely don't look forward to fires or hurricanes or tornados. As a matter of fact, most Americans spend huge sums of money on homeowners insurance over the years — insurance that is rarely needed.

- One of the newest forms of insurance that is growing in popularity deals with long-term care (LTC). This is far from inexpensive, but the security and peace of mind it offers is difficult to argue against. By definition it is coverage that provides nursing-home care, home-health care, personal or adult day care usually for individuals above the age of 65 or with a chronic or disabling condition that needs constant supervision. Today it is one of the most highly desired forms of insurance — but one that is often neglected.

Five examples of insurance that Americans spend billions of dollars on annually are strong indicators of the importance we place on protection.

Some people who have used this book over the years have actually referred to it as the "cheapest insurance they've ever acquired." Others have told me that ***The Me You Don't Know*** is a form of insurance that they really believe will be there for them and ready to go to work — not matter how many years down the road.

Strokes don't respect age. Certainly cancer doesn't. Multiple Sclerosis attacks the majority of its victims in their mid-twenties and thirties. We used to think Katherine Hepburn and Parkinson's in the same sentence — but Michael J. Fox certainly lowered the age ceiling. Alzheimer's was thought to be a disease that really attacked the elderly, but recent statistics indicate lower age groups showing initial stages. And how many of you are aware that there are nine forms of Muscular Dystrophy (not limited to just Jerry Lewis' Kids)? There are three forms that attack adults over the age of 50. I could illustrate more diseases and disabilities that have no respect for age, but the point has been made.

Once illness, disease, serious accident, or disability hits, once they impact an individual in such a serious way that they discover new words in their vocabulary — such as caregiver, it could be too late for the insurance that ***The Me You Don't Know*** could bring to their lives to be effective.

Regardless of caregiving being personalized or institutionalized, it is possible for any of us who allows ourselves to look into the future to help those who will eventually become our caregivers. We can help them understand us: who we are (now), who we were (when we were younger), what we like and dislike, what our hopes and desires for the future are, and how we want to have a say in how we are cared for down the road. If you take time now — before anything happens to drastically change your life (or changes it further) — it is possible that you can provide critically important information and data that future caregivers can put to use in order to provide a more positive and rewarding experience for you. You can have influence on your future caregiving. What an amazing concept.

The Me You Don't Know is more than a book. It is a tool — a tool that you can use to create a guide for those people who will one day have the responsibility of providing for you and assuring that your wishes and desires, your needs, and quality of life remain intact. But like any tool, it cannot do its job if it isn't put to work.

If you've purchased this book for yourself, congratulations. You've taken a very positive step. If you acquired this book for another person, you've just demonstrated a strong and valuable concern for their well being.

If you are the individual filling out the pages of this guide, I am sure that your future caregivers will appreciate your efforts. If you have acquired this book for someone else, rest assured that you are giving them something that they and their caregivers will find extremely valuable. However, if you are only giving this to someone else, I strongly urge you to fill one out for yourself. If you intend to help another person, why not help yourself as well?

In the first edition, I reprinted an article that Dee had read in *The Philadelphia Inquirer*. The author of the article, Dan Gottlieb, a clinical psychologist from Philadelphia, gave us permission to reprint his thoughts. The article is entitled:

A FATHER, A SON, AND A VACATION THAT WON'T BE FORGOTTEN

The following are excerpted portions:

Several years ago I never would have believed such a time could be filled with joy. That's because when my mother died in January 1998, my father was consumed with grief. After 56 years of being in a loving marriage, it was almost a year before he could hear her name without crying. His grief was raw and deep. But something good came out of the process. He and I were always close, but after her death we became even closer. For the first time in our relationship, he would share his sadness, regret and fear of the future.

Ever since I graduated from Atlantic City High School in 1964, I have dreamed about returning to the Shore for the summer. Despite my father's advancing age, I probably would have postponed my dream a few more years. But several months ago I learned that a friend of mine had died. This was a fellow quadriplegic — a man my age who had gone through rehabilitation with me. When his daughter informed me of his death, she said: "After 20 years as a quadriplegic, his body just gave out." I have been a quadriplegic for 22 years.

Later that day, I remembered a bumper sticker someone sent me years ago: "Don't postpone joy." So I called my father, who still lives in Atlantic City, and asked him how he felt about making his apartment wheelchair-accessible and spending the month of July with me. He was thrilled.

Over the course of the month we became roommates in every sense of the word. I teased him about his memory and he teased me when I left the screen door open and I hollered at him for being too rigid about time. We shared jokes, lunches, and we worried about each other.

But mostly we just talked. At the time, it seemed like what we talked about was not very important — where he was going to dinner, what television shows he liked, how he dealt with his insomnia, and various other chronic problems. But as I look back on those talks I realize that he was telling me about his life — the same way I told him about my life when I was in college.

Now I know that he religiously watches Jeopardy! When he is not out on a date. And that his brother calls at exactly 9 every morning. I know that he loves to read murder mysteries and always reads the last page first to make sure it has a happy ending. Little bits of information that seem trivial. As I leave the apartment, I have a picture of a day in his life. I also have other pictures etched in my memory from this vacation. I watched as he sat in his lounge chair holding his book 12 inches from his face, moving his head from side to side, drinking in each line. I watched as he slept in that same chair with the book in his lap. I watched as he sometimes stared out the window, lost in his own thoughts, his face reflecting whether he was thinking about his past or his future.

And I watched the animation as he spoke on the phone to one of his friends, and his loud laughter when he heard something funny or ribald. Each one of these observations felt like a snapshot in my mind that I pray will not fade when his chair is empty.

Best vacation I ever had.

Thanks, Dad

After reading Dan's article, the purpose of Dee Marella's guidebook became crystal clear. All the memories, the great stories, the mental images — that's all that we will have left. What about the basic facts of our lives? If only some of them had been written down.

This is one of the reasons that this guide is so very important. It provides a stimulus that we all need to set down in writing — the thoughts and memories, the needs and desires that our future caregivers will use to serve us better. This is a golden opportunity to actually speak into the future — when, perhaps we cannot speak for ourselves.

It is my sincere hope that each person who picks up a copy of ***The Me You Don't Know*** will be inspired to put down in writing those seemingly-insignificant or trivial facts and bits of data about themselves so that one day those words might make all the difference in the world to a caregiver who reads them — and to YOU.

— **Dennis McClellan**
Publisher

PART I

For Caregivers

The first section of this book is directed to those people — family, friends, and strangers — who will serve as my caregivers sometime in the future. When you read through these pages, keep in mind that I have made sincere efforts to help you understand me, but I've also attempted to understand you, my caregivers, and the important role you will play in my life in the future. Thanks in advance.

A PERSONAL NOTE TO MY FUTURE CAREGIVERS

WHEN I AM IN NEED OF YOUR CARE, I realize there will be times when I will exasperate you, and you will get annoyed with my table manners, forgetfulness, etc. Your responsibilities while caring for me will sometimes seem overwhelming. Any "tool" I can give you to help you function more effectively will make me feel better.

Signature ______________________

TOP 10 PRIORITIES FOR CAREGIVERS

This list is adapted from the personal experiences of a caregiver.

1) LOVE

If you can do something to make someone more comfortable, do it! Don't have regrets when they are gone.

2) ASSURANCE

Do your best and that is all anyone can ask of you. Don't compare notes with siblings, it only causes strife and tension.

3) PEACE OF MIND

If your loved one is in a nursing home, go at various times of the day to visit. This way you can see for yourself if your loved one Is being cared for adequately at all times.

4) COMFORT

Don't give "goodies" to a loved one when you come to visit. Your time and loving attention are what is needed when you arrive. Give the "goodies" to them when you are leaving. By doing so, you see your loved one occupied and content when you are leaving.

5) INFORMATION

Find out the wishes and desires of the loved one you are caring for. Don't assume you know. Talk TO him/her, don't talk AT them.

6) COMRADESHIP

Find a cherished friend or confidant to use as a sounding board. You are giving your time, efforts and love as a caregiver. Don't diminish your efforts by complaining to everyone you meet.

7) FAITH

If you are open to this, lean on your faith during a very trying time. My faith and hope truly pulled me through.

8) BALANCE

Take care of yourself. You NEED an outlet. If you are uptight and stressed, you will pass this onto your family and the loved one you are caring for.

9) KNOWLEDGE

Know that you are not alone during this trying time. Use the resources available, (i.e. support groups, Internet resources, clergy, and other caregivers.)

10) ACCEPTANCE

You are only one human being. You cannot make a person healthy or happy... you can only try to make him/her comfortable. When you have done all that you can, no more should be expected of you.

GENERAL GUIDANCE FOR MY FUTURE CAREGIVERS

Please help see that:

- I will be kept clean.
- I will be fed nutritious meals.
- I will be helped to keep my dignity as much as possible.
- I will obtain necessary medical care.
- I will not be treated as though I am already dead. I hope I will have the opportunity to continue to be around things I love — family, friends, jokes, music, movies, and good food until the day I do die!!
- I hope to be remembered for the love and support I tried to give to my family and friends. To be loved in return is to have true wealth.

While I am still "rational," I do realize that later:

- You cannot be with me 24 hours a day.
- You must go on with your life.
- You love me and will try to do your best to help keep me comfortable.

- At times, you will feel anger and guilt when I thrash out in frustration. I am not angry with you. I am angry and frustrated that I have become helpless.
- You did not make me sick.
- You must take care of your family and yourself. Don't feel guilty when you cannot be with me. Go on with your life.

Thank you in advance for the care and comfort you will offer.

Signed: ______________________________

THINGS I LEARNED WHEN I WAS A CAREGIVER

A Note to My Future Caregivers

SINCE YOU ARE THE ONE who will be in need of care in the future, feel free to add anything you feel appropriate. If you disagree with something, cross it out. This guide must become "your guide."

If you have brothers or sisters, ***do not*** expect every one of them to take care of your parent in the same way. Each person has to live with his/her own decisions. Each should pretend he/she is ***an only child***. Do not compare notes about what each one is doing or not doing. It only leads to anger, family strife and illness. You do what you can — with love.

Do not look for praise or condemnation. It is to God that you have to answer. If you truly believe you are doing your share to help care and give your loved one love and kindness, so be it.

It is so much easier to care for a loved one when everyone ***cooperates***. Talk together. Plan together. Just don't compare!

When you visit an incapacitated person, give him/her your ***undivided attention***. Do not always look rushed and frustrated. Sometime you might be the only visitor he/she sees for days. A hug, kiss and sincere smile means so much. Sit close and hold his/her hand. ***Show*** the love you feel.

Before each visit, take a minute to visualize yourself in the condition and environment. What would be ***your*** physical and emotional needs?

Do not ***talk down*** to the person for whom you are providing care.

Take the person out of their environment as much as possible. Let him/her feel alive. A mall is a great place to go. (People to watch, varieties of food, accommodations for wheelchairs, and bathrooms are accessible.) Such small "outings" will let the person know his/her "confinement" will not be continuous.

If possible, bring a favorite food when you visit. For an extra special treat, set a pretty table with flowers, etc. Bring an up-to-date album to show the latest family pictures.

Carry a comb, makeup, nail polish, etc. with you if you are visiting. If the person you are visiting is male, why not surprise him with his favorite aftershave or cologne?

Before I would leave, I always handed my Mom a newspaper, magazine or something I knew she enjoyed. That way, she had something to look forward to when I left. Leave with a big hug and a promise to return.

Each time I would leave, I told my Mom something she could look forward to when I came back. "Mom, Tuesday we will visit Peggy. Mom, I am bringing Alice to visit with you on Thursday. Mom, I am taking you to the shore on Monday and Tuesday." Everyone needs a reason to go on living.

Treat your loved one the way you would want to be treated.

Do not kid yourself into thinking your own children are not watching. They are observing how lovingly you treat your Mom and Dad or other family members. More often than not, that is the way you will be treated someday.

Be fair, loving, kind, and compassionate. Keep calm, but stay in control.

GIFTS FOR THOSE BEING CARED FOR AND IDEAS FOR CAREGIVERS, FAMILY AND FRIENDS

- To pay bills or run errands for your care recipient, have him/her put all bills and list of needs into one box. You can pick these up when you visit.
- Leave a few dollars so that a pizza can be ordered or some other special treat.
- If the person is in a wheelchair, clip a portable digital phone to the chair. (Purchase one that has 1-button-dialing for often-used numbers.)
- Purchase a clock with large numerals for the wall.
- Purchase a calendar with large squares and fill in important family dates: birthdays, anniversaries, etc.
- Purchase a bulletin board and attach recent pictures of the family.
- Frame and hang a picture of the care recipient over his/her bed. A picture taken when he/she was young and vibrant.

- Check and see that he/she has an adequate supply of allowed snacks.
- Purchase a radio and put it on a station he/she likes to listen to. (Then, only the "ON"/ "OFF" knob has to be turned to "ON.")
- Purchase a beautiful notebook for visitors to sign. (This even helps the caregiver to check on who has been in for a visit.)
- Foster closeness by giving your loved one a weekly manicure. It provides "private time" to talk and to make personal contact with one another.
- If your care recipient is living at home alone, make certain all medicines can easily be opened. Write out IN BIG LETTERS the quantities and times each medication must be taken.
- Help remove facial hair – this is a constant concern for both women and men.
- Make certain hair is always washed and well groomed.
- Do not visit at the same time if your loved one is in a nursing home. Check in at different and varied times to make certain your loved one is getting proper care all day long — not just during anticipated visits.

PERSONAL BELIEFS
What I Have Learned in Life

FOR CAREGIVERS

A LETTER TO MY FUTURE CAREGIVERS

THE FOLLOWING LETTER WAS written to my three daughters, Tammy, Lani and Robin. I wrote it with love. It will go inside my personal copy of *The Me You Don't Know*.

Write a similar letter now, while you are able to convey your true feelings. Do not worry about spelling or grammar. Just say what is in your heart. It will mean so much later on. Just do it!

Dear Tammy, Lani and Robin,

One of my deepest fears is the thought of one day growing old and helpless. I pray that God takes me first. However, there is a strong possibility that He will not. In that case, I want to make the burden of your caring for me as easy and gentle as possible.

When Grandmom became "dead weight" and she had to enter a nursing home, I think you can remember how much it broke my heart. She always asked my sisters and me to promise never to put her into a nursing home. I promised, with sincere, loving intentions — but could not keep my promise when she was beyond my physical and mental capabilities. I never want any of you to proclaim that you would never put your mother or father in a nursing home. Sometimes it will be beyond your control. All I ask is that you research and find a home that "feels right" for me. Is the staff friendly? Do the residents look clean and content? Are there visitors around? If possible, I would like a private room. (You know how I react to bad odors, etc.) Please keep air fresheners and potpourri in my room.

When you come to visit, please don't tell me you can't stay very long. That tells me you are there because of obligation. Truthfully, in that case, I would rather you stay away and get whatever is rushing you out of the way. Just come and see me when you can spend quality time holding my hand, talking to me and seeing that I am okay. I say all of the above with love and understanding — not with anger.

Remember that your husband and children take priority. I know what it was like juggling children's activities, meals, household necessities, husband's needs, and to worry and feel guilty about my sick mother. Remember when Grandmom Bea was in the nursing home? I was living in Pennsylvania. Your Dad and I decided that I would leave Pennsylvania every Monday morning and spend Monday and Tuesday in New Jersey with Grandmom. I would pick her up at 9:30 AM and take her back at 4 PM. Each day I would try to plan to have some of her friends meet us at the mall. This sometimes became difficult because she was 91 and most of her friends had passed away. Anyway, by Tuesday at 4 PM, when I dropped her off before heading back to PA, I was exhausted and filled with guilt about having to leave her. I never left her once when she said, "Thank you for coming. I had a nice time. I'll see you next time." She would always look depressed and would say, "Why do you always have to leave so soon?" I realized she didn't want to be where she was. She was always such an alive, active person. I would drive home crying and feeling guilty. I never want you girls to feel that way. I thank you, from the bottom of my heart, for any quality time you will give me in the future. Never feel guilty when you have to leave.

If I am visiting in your home, please talk to me. I may get deaf and I might have weak eyesight, but I can cope with these. I could not cope, however, with being tolerated or forgotten. I desire to be a viable member of the family. I want my grandchildren to love me and want to be around me. Laughter is such a healer. It bothers me so much to see older people sitting amongst others and just listening and not joining in. (Do they feel left out? Do they not want to interact? What makes them feel this way?)

Tammy, Lani and Robin — I want to thank you for being such wonderful daughters. You have always been there when Dad and I needed you. When you heard about Dad's heart operation, Tammy, you organized a schedule so that each of you would spend one week with me. By the end of three weeks, Dad was well on his way to recovery. Lani and Robin — remember when you got the initial call saying Dad had his heart attack? You came right to the hospital in Pennsylvania from New Jersey without packing or grabbing your purses. That shows how little you thought of yourselves at a time when you were needed.

Very often a little old lady sat in a wheelchair by the main entry to Grandmom's nursing home. I would give her a big greeting and hug each time I saw her. One day she grabbed my arm and pulled me back. She said, "I want you to promise to remember what I am going to tell you. When they put me in this nursing home, they took away my house, my car, my furniture — but they couldn't take away my memories. Go out and get as many good memories as you can."

Tammy, Lani and Robin — thank you for being such loving daughters. I have many wonderful, happy memories of times shared with you. I love you!

— **Mom**

PS: Always take care of each other.

PERSONAL LETTER TO MY FUTURE CAREGIVERS

Date: ______________________________

Dear: ______________________________

PART II

My Healthcare

The following section is a critically important part of this guidebook. Please take care to put accurate information onto each page. Don't hesitate to make changes, should that be required in the future. What is written here today may not be accurate five years from now. Here you will enter information, for example, about your medical history, the medications you take, healthcare professionals that you work with, and those you never want to go back to.

PRIORITIES FOR CARE

Address each section as completely as possible. If possible, fill this part out with pencil for ease of updating.

> **NOTE:** Update this section whenever there is a change in medication, attending physicians, etc.

Making medical decisions for an incompetent loved one can be an anguishing task for a caretaker.

MY PREFERRED HEALTHCARE PROVIDERS/AGENTS

Physician:

Name

Phone

Address

Dentist:

Name

Phone

Address

Podiatrist:

Name

Phone

Address

Optometrist:

Name

Phone

Address

Optician: Name ______________________
Phone ______________________
Address ______________________
____

Pharmacy: Name ______________________
Phone ______________________
Address ______________________
____

Hospital: Name ______________________
Phone ______________________
Address ______________________
____

Insurance Agent: Name ______________________
Phone ______________________
Address ______________________
____

Insurance Agent: Name ______________________
Phone ______________________
Address ______________________
____

Other: Name ______________________
Phone ______________________
Address ______________________
____

DOCTORS, HOSPITALS, OTHER PROFESSIONALS THAT *I NEVER WANT TO GO BACK* TO

Name ______________________________

Phone ______________________________

Address ______________________________

____

Name ______________________________

Phone ______________________________

Address ______________________________

____

Name ______________________________

Phone ______________________________

Address ______________________________

PERSONAL MEDICAL HISTORY

The following is a list of known medical conditions/major injuries that should be noted:

Name of illness/injury:

Age of occurrence: ____________________

Type of treatment: ____________________

Long-term impact: ____________________

Name of illness/injury:

Age of occurrence: ____________________

Type of treatment: ____________________

Long-term impact: ____________________

Name of illness/injury:

Age of occurrence:

Type of treatment:

Long-term impact:

Name of illness/injury:

Age of occurrence:

Type of treatment:

Long-term impact:

Name of illness/injury:

Age of occurrence:

Type of treatment:

Long-term impact:

Name of illness/injury:

Age of occurrence: ______

Type of treatment: ______

Long-term impact: ______

Name of illness/injury:

Age of occurrence: ______

Type of treatment: ______

Long-term impact: ______

Name of illness/injury:

Age of occurrence: ______

Type of treatment: ______

Long-term impact: ______

Physical problems I have and medications I take for them (include all prescription and over-the-counter drugs):

Allergies I have and medications I take for them (include all prescription and across-the-counter drugs):

My family history of reproductive problems (miscarriages, stillbirths, infertility, birth defects):

My family history of diseases (diabetes, cardiac, mental challenges, etc.):

EMERGENCY CONTACTS

(Copy this page and place it on refrigerator or any other obvious place)

Family member ____________________

Cell Phone # ____________________

Doctor ____________________

Cell Phone # ____________________

Hospital ____________________

Cell Phone # ____________________

Police (Nonemergency) ____________________

Cell Phone # ____________________

Emergency 911 ____________________

Veterinarian ____________________

Cell Phone # ____________________

Pharmacy ____________________

Cell Phone # ____________________

Alarm Company ____________________

Cell Phone # ____________________

Location of ***The Me You Don't Know*** for further vital information:

____

____

____

____

IF I HAD A TERMINAL ILLNESS

_______ I would want to know.

_______ I would not want to know.

Comments on above:

Would I want you to request any hospital or doctor to keep me alive through extreme means if I were suffering?

______ **Yes** ______ **No**

My feelings on the use heroic measures and life support:

LIVING WILL

A LIVING WILL IS A DOCUMENT (also known as an advanced directive) that states in prior to a serious illness or accident what medical treatments you want or don't want to receive. It can also be a document in which the signer requests to be allowed to die rather than be kept alive by artificial means if disabled beyond a reasonable expectation of recovery. When signed by a competent person, it can provide guidance for medical and health-care decisions (as the termination of life support or organ donation) in the event the person becomes incompetent to make such decisions.

> For samples of living wills and powers of attorney, please look at the appendix on pages 217 – 228.
>
> While it is the intention of the publisher to alert users to their options in preparing for the future, please note that DC Press does not offer legal, medical or accounting advice Prior to attempting to utilize any form presented in this book or when making an important decision effecting your future healthcare or finances, seek the advise of a legal, accounting, and/or medical professionals.

A simple statement could be created and signed in front of witnesses. It is recommended that two witnesses also sign the document. Those witnesses should not be direct members of your family or someone who would benefit financially in the event of your death.

NOTE: It is very important to understand that if you fail to make a living will accessible to others, it is actually of no value and becomes completely worthless. Copies of your living will should be (1) kept with this guide and (2) given to any member of your immediate family that you feel should have one, (3) to your primary care physician and any specialists you work with, (4) your attorney, (5) and the hospital to which you feel you would most likely be taken in case of an emergency. If you are admitted to a nursing home, make sure the administration has a copy. It wouldn't be a bad idea to carry a copy in your purse or wallet.

Always discuss any matters of a legal nature with an attorney of your choice.

> *Many people today are worried about the medical care they would be given if they should become terminally ill and unable to communicate. They don't want to spend months or years dependent on life-supporting machines, and they don't want to cause unnecessary emotional or financial stress for their loved ones.*
>
> —**American Hospital Association**
> "Put It in Writing: Questions and Answers or Advance Directives"

I want the following to be done:

- If my heart stops, I do ____ do not ____ want CPR (cardio-pulmonary resuscitation).

- I do ____ do not ____ want to be placed on any mechanical breathing apparatus.

- I do ____ do not ____ wish to have any blood transfusions.

- I do ____ do not ____ want any intravenous food administered.

- I do ____ do not ____ want any liquids administered intravenously.

- If I am transported to a healthcare facility and placed on life support, I do ____ do not ____ want it stopped at the directive of my representative(s).

Comments on this subject:

- ______________________________

____

____

____

____

____

____

I Would Like to Be an Organ Donor:

_____ Yes _____ No

Comments on Organ Donation:

Any Special Requests Regarding Organ Donation:

MY THOUGHTS ON NURSING HOMES OR ASSISTED LIVING FACILITIES

PLANS I HAVE MADE*

Name of facility: ______________________________

Address: ______________________________

____

____

Phone: ______________________________

Contact Person: ______________________________

e-mail: ______________________________

cell phone: ______________________________

Additional Comments: ______________________________

____

____

____

____

____

*See page175 for Long-Term Healthcare Policy Information

CARING FOR MY PETS IN A TIME OF EMERGENCY

PET#1

Type of pet: ______________________________

Name of pet: ______________________________

Pet named ____________, does NOT like the following (thought it important to let you know): ______________________________

____

Specific Health Issues: ______________________________

____

____

Medications: ______________________________

____

Location of Vaccination Information: ______________________________

____

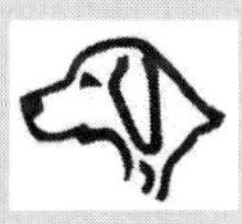

Suggestion: Consider placing your cell phone number on your pet's collar."

PET#2

Type of pet: ______________________________

Name of pet: ______________________________

Pet named ____________, does NOT like the following (thought it important to let you know): ____________________

Specific Health Issues: ____________________

Medications: ____________________

Location of Vaccination Information: ____________________

PET#3

Type of pet: ____________________

Name of pet: ____________________

Pet named _____________, does NOT like the following (thought it important to let you know): ____________________

Specific Health Issues: ____________________

Medications: ____________________

Location of Vaccination Information: ____________________

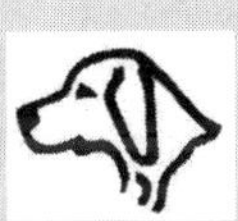

Suggestion: Any papers/proof that pets have current vaccinations should be kept in a folder/large envelope and clearly marked."

Veterinarian: Name ____________________

Phone ____________________

Address ____________________

____

Pet Groomer: Name ____________________

Phone ____________________

Address ____________________

____

Kennel: Name ____________________

Phone ____________________

Address ____________________

____

Name and telephone number of individual who could care for pet temporarily:

Name ____________________

Phone ____________________

Address ____________________

____

Brand of General Pet Food:

Dry ____________________

____

Wet ____________________

____

Brand of Biscuits: ____________________

Brand of Special Treats: ____________________

Exercise habits: ______________________________

____

____

Where he/she prefers to sleep: ______________________________

____

____

Would you like your pet to visit you if possible?

_____ Yes _____ No

Arrangements for permanent care for my pet — to assure that my pet is loved and properly cared for:

____

____

____

____

____

____

____

____

____

____

____

____

PART IV

My Preferences

If you understand my health and medical status, you know just one aspect of who I am. I have many things that I like, some that I dislike, and some things that I want nothing to do with. There are tastes and smell, sounds and images, colors, books and movies, and so many other things that really describe who I am. When you read the following, please know that I've given lots of thought to what is written here. I believe these bits of information about me will help you understand the real me.

WHO AM I?

It is important you understand my innermost feelings and I feel about myself. Do you know the things about myself that I like and things I dislike? How about the world around me?

I realize that there are no "right" or "wrong" responses when describing my feelings. I've taken into consideration the following examples provided by the author — but realize they are only "examples."

- I am very "thin skinned." My feelings can get hurt very easily. Because I am this way, I try to "feel" for others and not offend them.
- I believe every child should get a fine education. Equally important, however, I believe every child should be taught the importance of manners and honesty — or you, as a parent, have "shortchanged" your child.
- God gave each of us special talents. It is a sin if you do not use these talents to make the world a better place.
- One of the most evil things on this earth is prejudice. I try to look each person squarely in the eye and decide if I like or dislike what I see. I think it is so wrong to judge a person because of his/her color, religion or nationality. We could learn so much from each other.

Important fact to know about me:

I prefer to do things by myself ______

I prefer to work with others ______

List of my innermost likes and dislikes — about myself and the world around me.

FEARS I HAVE

I am sharing my personal fears with you, my future caregivers. I believe it important to note that I understand there is no set number of "correct" responses. And I understand that the following are merely "examples" the author has provided."

- I am not afraid of death. I am afraid of pain and suffering. Medicate me, even if it means a shorter life
- Being treated like a child in my later life is a fear I have. Please never talk down to me or "pat me on the head." Allow me to keep my dignity.
- Make certain that I am never fed anything with a Red Sauce or Mayonnaise. I gag on both.
- I am very shy. If possible, please do not let a male nurse care for me.
- I fear strife in the family if Dad or I were alone and sickly. Our family has such love and closeness now. Please do not let Dad or me cause that to change. Work together. Try to keep a sense of humor. Two things have always helped me when things got really stressful with Gram: faith in God and a good laugh.

Fears I Have and How I Handle Them:

FAVORITE PRODUCT BRANDS

Toothpaste: __________

Mouthwash: __________

Laxative: __________

Headache Remedy: __________

Vitamins:

General Multivitamin: __________

Vitamin C: __________

Other: __________

Other: __________

Other: __________

Deodorant: __________

Perfume/Cologne/Aftershave Lotion: __________

Lipstick Color: __________

Makeup:

1. ____________________
2. ____________________
3. ____________________

Hair Coloring Kit: ____________________

Hairspray: ____________________

Nail Polish: ____________________

Moisturizer: ____________________

Razor: ____________________

Shaving Cream: ____________________

Facial Hair Remover: ____________________

Soap: ____________________

Beauty Salon:

Name: ____________________

Address: ____________________

Phone: ____________________

Barber:

Name: ____________________

Address: ____________________

Phone: ____________________

Other Items:

Products that cause sensitivity and/or allergic reactions:

Additional information that you should know about how I prefer to maintain myself cosmetically:

CLOTHING PREFERENCES

CLOTHING SIZES

Female	Male
_______ Dress	_______ Suit
_______ Blouse	_______ Shirt
_______ Slacks	_______ Trousers
_______ Outer Coat	_______ Outer Coat
_______ Sweater	_______ Sweater
_______ Shoes	_______ Shoes
_______ Stockings	_______ Socks
_______ Pajamas	_______ Pajamas
_______ Nightgown	
_______ Slippers	_______ Slippers
_______ Housecoat	_______ Robe
_______ Slips	Underwear
_______ Underpants	_______ T-Shirts
_______ Bras	_______ Shorts
	_______ Boxers
	_______ Briefs

Bedtime clothing I feel most comfortable wearing (Put in order of favorites — "1" being my favorite):

_____ Nightgown

_____ Pajamas

_____ Underwear

_____ Other

My Favorite Bed Pillow: (Check one)

_____ Soft

_____ Medium

_____ Hard

I like to take: (Check one)

_____ Showers

_____ Baths

Comments on Above:

Clothes I am most comfortable in:

Clothes I do not like to wear:

My favorite colors to wear:

Three favorite outfits I like to wear:

1.

2.

3.

If given one small closet and one dresser, the following is what I would choose to put in these places. If I had to sort through all my clothes, jewelry, books, and other possessions today, here are the most important items.

FOOD PREFERENCES

For Breakfast:

For Lunch:

For Dinner:

Foods I love and would eat at any time:

Foods I absolutely hate and would never eat:

Foods I am allergic to:

My favorite snack foods include:

My thoughts on organic food:

My favorite soups are:

My favorite salads and dressings include:

My favorite entrees are:

My favorite:

Candy:

Cake:

Pie:

Ice Cream:

Ethnic foods I do/do not enjoy:

Family recipes I enjoy: Here are complete recipes that I've created, make regularly, or are familiar to family members. (Attach a memory that goes along with each recipe.)

MY TALENTS AND INTERESTS

- Musical Instruments I play (or played):

- Singing Ability:

- Acting Ability:

Hobbies:

Other Interests/Talents/Skills:

ENTERTAINMENT PREFERENCES

Types of TV shows I enjoy:

Favorite movies and videos I enjoy viewing:

Favorite TV channels:

Sports I like to watch (on TV or in person):

Sport	Favorite Team

Favorite TV stars:

Favorite movie stars:

Types of TV shows / Movies that I do not enjoy:

Radio programs I enjoy:

Radio programs I do not enjoy:

Music I enjoy listening to:

Music that gives me a headache:

Favorite singers:

Newspapers and Magazines I enjoy reading:

My favorite authors:

My favorite religious passages, scriptures, meditations, readings:

Card games I enjoy:

Board games I enjoy:

My favorite websites:

PLACES I LIKE TO VISIT

Where I like to go for drives in the car:

For Breakfast (name restaurants):

For Lunch (name restaurants):

For Dinner (name restaurants):

For Sightseeing/Historic Landmarks:

Museums/Libaries/Theaters:

IF I AM INVITED OUT FOR A DAY OR EVENING, THIS IS WHAT I WOULD LIKE TO DO

In town:

Out of town:

PEOPLE I ALWAYS ENJOY SEEING

Name

Phone

Cell Phone

E-mail Address:

Address

Name

Phone

Cell Phone

E-mail Address:

Address

Name ____________________

Phone ____________________

Cell Phone ____________________

E-mail Address: ____________________

Address ____________________

____

Name ____________________

Phone ____________________

Cell Phone ____________________

E-mail Address: ____________________

Address ____________________

____

Name ____________________

Cell Phone ____________________

Phone ____________________

E-mail Address: ____________________

Address ____________________

____

If additional names should be included, place the information on page 233 (NOTES).

MY TYPICAL DAY

I think it important for any caregiver to understand what my typical day is like and how much it means that these routine activities and rituals be maintained as much as possible.

- **I am a __ day person __ night person. (Check proper response.)**
- **I usually wake at ________ AM.**
- **I like eating breakfast at ________ AM.**
- **Most mornings I enjoy: (examples: reading, gardening, watching TV, e-mailing friends)**

  ____

  ____

- **I like to eat my lunch at ________ AM or PM.**
- **I enjoy an afternoon nap at ________ PM.**
- **Most afternoons I enjoy:**

  ____

  ____

- I like to eat dinner at ______________ PM.
- After dinner I enjoy:

____

____

____

____

____

- I usually get ready for bed at ______________ PM.
- I like to:

Read in bed ________

Watch TV in bed ________

Go right to sleep ________

- I communicate daily with the following people:

Name ______________________________

Relationship ______________________________

Phone # ______________________________

E-mail address ______________________________

Name ______________________________

Relationship ______________________________

Phone # ______________________________

E-mail address ______________________________

Name

Relationship

Phone #

E-mail address

Name

Relationship

Phone #

E-mail address

Name

Relationship

Phone #

E-mail address

Name

Relationship

Phone #

E-mail address

Name

Relationship

Phone #

E-mail address

RELIGIOUS AFFILIATION

Church, Synagogue, Mosque, Religious Facility:

Address:

Telephone #:

e-mail:

Web Site:

Key Contact Person(s):

Name:

Cell Phone:

Describe Attendance (include time of day, seating area, and other important points):

Describe Participation (such as choir, usher, teacher, etc.):

The importance of religion in my life:

The importance of faith at the time of my death:

PREFERRED FUNERAL ARRANGEMENTS

Funeral Home

Name ______________________________

Phone ______________________________

Address ______________________________

____

I would like to be:

______ Buried/Placed in Mausoleum

Location ______________________

City / State ______________________

______ Cremated

Location ______________________

City / State ______________________

Note: if any prior arrangements have been made, where can those documents be located, including plans for ashes if cremated:

____

____

I would like to wear the color(s):

____

____

I would like this church/temple/place of worship to be used for the ceremony (name of location, city):

Location ______________________________

City / State ______________________________

I would like this Priest, Rabbi, or Clergyman to preside over the ceremony:

Name ______________________________

Phone ______________________________

Address ______________________________

____

I would like the following Funeral Home and Funeral Director:

Name ______________________________

Phone ______________________________

Address ______________________________

____

Lodge or Military Affiliation to be contacted:

Name ______________________________

Phone ______________________________

Address ______________________________

____

In lieu of flowers:

I would like the following flowers:

I would like the following music played at the place of worship:

I would like these prayers said at my funeral:

I would like to have the following inscribed on my tombstone or grave marker:

____

____

____

I would like the following donations made in my memory (list organizations, groups, individuals):

____

____

____

I want these items placed in the coffin with me:

____

____

____

I would prefer "at the viewing":

____An open casket ____A closed casket

____No viewing

____I prefer a memorial service rather than a viewing

____Casket or cremation vessel present

____No Casket or cremation vessel present

Pallbearer preferences:

Name ______

Phone ______

Cell Phone ______

E-mail Address: ______

Address ______

______

Name ______

Phone ______

Cell Phone ______

E-mail Address: ______

Address ______

______

Name ______

Phone ______

Cell Phone ______

E-mail Address: ______

Address ______

______

Name ______

Phone ______

Cell Phone ______

E-mail Address: ______

Address ______

______

I would like the following included in my obituary:

REGRETS IN MY LIFE

If I had to do it all over again...

Regrets I Have:

Special interests I wish I had pursued:

What is really important in life:

PART V

My Finances

My financial information is obviously important and highly personal. What I provide on the following pages is intended to aid and assist those who are caring for me. I appreciate that this information is respected and used only for the purpose of making my life better.

IMPORTANT NAMES AND PHONE NUMBERS

Important Names and Phone Numbers (this list includes individuals you deal with both personally and for business):

Bank

Name ______

Phone ______

Address ______

______

List all account numbers ______

______

______

______

______

Financial Planner

Name ______

Phone ______

Address ______

______

Attorney

Name ______________________________

Phone ______________________________

Address ______________________________

____

Accountant

Name ______________________________

Phone ______________________________

Address ______________________________

____

Tax Preparer

Name ______________________________

Phone ______________________________

Address ______________________________

____

Location of Previous Tax Records

Name ______________________________

Phone ______________________________

Address ______________________________

____

Broker

Name

Phone

Address

Money Market Fund

Name

Phone

Address

Account Number(s)

Name

Phone

Address

Account Number(s)

Name

Phone

Address

Account Number(s)

IRAs

Name

Phone

Address

Account Number(s)

Name

Phone

Address

Account Number(s)

Funeral Home

Name

Phone

Address

Safety Deposit Box/Keys

Name

Phone

Address

Box Number

MY PERSONAL & BUSINESS AFFAIRS

Locating and understanding where important papers can be found (provide location, contact person if needed, contact phone numbers):

Original Will:

Name of Attorney ____________________

Phone ____________________

Address ____________________

Executor(s) of Will:

Name of Attorney ____________________

Phone ____________________

Address ____________________

Name of Attorney ____________________

Phone ____________________

Address ____________________

Powers of Attorney (If different than above):

Name of Attorney ____________________

Phone ____________________

Address ____________________

Name of Attorney ____________________

Phone ____________________

Address ____________________

Copies of Will:

Name ____________________

Phone ____________________

Address ____________________

Name ____________________

Phone ____________________

Address ____________________

Trusts:

Location ____________________

Type ____________________

Name of Trustee ____________________

Address ____________________

Phone ____________________

Checking Account(s):

Name ____________________

Phone ____________________

Address ____________________

Account Number(s) ____________________

Savings Account(s):

Name ____________________

Phone ____________________

Address ____________________

Account Number(s) ____________________

Real Estate (Deeds, Mortgages, Rental Agreements)

Name/Location ______________________

Phone ______________________

Address ______________________

____

Contact ______________________

Titles (Automobile and Other Vehicles)

Name/Location ______________________

Phone ______________________

Address ______________________

____

Contact ______________________

IRAs

Name ______________________

Phone ______________________

Address ______________________

____

Account Number(s) ______________________

Stock Certificates:

Name ______

Phone ______

Address ______

Owner's Name ______

Name ______

Phone ______

Address ______

______

Owner's Name ______

Name ______

Phone ______

Address ______

______

Owner's Name ______

Name ______

Phone ______

Address ______

______

Owner's Name ______

Bonds:

Name ______

Address ______

______

Phone ______

Owner's Name ______

Name ______

Address ______

______

Phone ______

Owner's Name ______

Name ______

Address ______

______

Phone ______

Owner's Name ______

Name ______

Address ______

______

Phone ______

Owner's Name ______

INSURANCE POLICIES

Life Insurance

Name of Insurance Company

Insurance Company Phone #

Policy #

Group#

Member ID# (If Applicable)

Co-pays# (If Applicable)

Address of Company

Location of Policy

House/Real Estate/Rental Property Insurance:

Name of Insurance Company

Insurance Company Phone #

Policy #

Group#

Member ID# (If Applicable)

Co-pays# (If Applicable)

Address of Company

Location of Policy

Automotive Insurance:

Name of Insurance Company ______________________

Insurance Company Phone # ______________________

Policy # ______________________

Group# ______________________

Member ID# (If Applicable) ______________________

Co-pays# (If Applicable) ______________________

Address of Company ______________________

____

Location of Policy ______________________

Health Insurance:

Name of Insurance Company ______________________

Insurance Company Phone # ______________________

Policy # ______________________

Group# ______________________

Member ID# (If Applicable) ______________________

Co-pays# (If Applicable) ______________________

Address of Company ______________________

____

Location of Policy ______________________

Dental Insurance:

Name of Insurance Company ____________________

Insurance Company Phone # ____________________

Policy # ____________________

Group# ____________________

Member ID# (If Applicable) ____________________

Co-pays# (If Applicable) ____________________

Address of Company ____________________

____

Location of Policy ____________________

Vision Insurance:

Name of Insurance Company ____________________

Insurance Company Phone # ____________________

Policy # ____________________

Group# ____________________

Member ID# (If Applicable) ____________________

Co-pays# (If Applicable) ____________________

Address of Company ____________________

____

Location of Policy ____________________

Long-Term Health Insurance:

Name of Insurance Company ____________________

Insurance Company Phone # ____________________

Policy # ____________________

Group# ____________________

Member ID# (If Applicable) ____________________

Co-pays# (If Applicable) ____________________

Address of Company ____________________

____

Location of Policy ____________________

Cash or Long-Term Care Policy that I have to cover costs:

Name of Policy ____________________

Policy # ____________________

Address of Carrier ____________________

Location of Policy ____________________

Dedicated Cash Account:

Location ____________________

Contact ____________________

Address ____________________

Phone ____________________

Comments ____________________

PENSIONS & RETIREMENT ACCOUNTS

Title of Pension Plan/Retirement Account:

____

Account Number: ______________________________

Location: ______________________________

Title of Pension Plan/Retirement Account:

____

Account Number: ______________________________

Location: ______________________________

Title of Pension Plan/Retirement Account:

____

Account Number: ______________________________

Location: ______________________________

401(k):

Name ______________________________

Address ______________________________

Phone ______________________________

Owner's Name ______________________________

Location: ______________________________

Non-bank IRAs:

Name

Address

Phone

Owner's Name

Social Security Information:

Number:

Location:

Notes:

MILITARY RETIREMENT BENEFITS

Military Branch: ____________________

Military ID Number: ____________________

Duration of Service: From: __________ To: __________

From: __________ To: __________

Discharge Date: ____________________

BENEFITS:

VA Pension: Veterans Pension: ____________________

Spouse & Child Pension: ____________________

VA Disability Compensation: ____________________

Combat Related Special Compensation: ____________________

Burial Benefits: ____________________

Survivor & Dependents Benefits: ____________________

Servicemembers' Benefits: ____________________

Veterans' Life Insurance: ____________________

Location of Military Papers: ____________________

MEDICARE

Medicare Information:

Number: ______________________________

Notes: ______________________________

____

Medicaid Information:

Number: ______________________________

Notes: ______________________________

____

Medicare Rx Info:

Number: ______________________________

Notes: ______________________________

____

Medicare Supplemental Info:

Notes: ______________________________

____

____

SPECIAL COLLECTIONS

(i.e., stamps, coins, other collectables)

Item #1 Name: ______________________

Notes: ______________________

____

____

____

Name ______________________

Address ______________________

____

Phone ______________________

Item #2 Name: ______________________

Notes: ______________________

____

____

____

Name ______________________

Address ______________________

____

Phone ______________________

Item #3 Name: ______________________

Notes: ______________________

____

Name ______________________

Address ______________________

____

Phone ______________________

Item #4 Name: ______________________

Notes: ______________________

____

Name ______________________

Address ______________________

____

Phone ______________________

Item #5 Name: ______________________

Notes: ______________________

____

Name ______________________

Address ______________________

____

Phone ______________________

INHERITANCE

Explain the details of any inheritance due:

LIST OF ASSETS

Home:

Address: ____________________

Purchase Price: ____________________

Current Value: ____________________

Date of last appraisal: ____________________

Location of Deed(s): ____________________

Automobile(s):

Make/Model: ____________________

Year: ____________________

Location of Title: ____________________

Make/Model: ____________________

Year: ____________________

Location of Title: ____________________

Make/Model: ____________________

Year: ____________________

Location of Title: ____________________

Recreational Vehicles (Boats, Trailers, Jet Skis, Snow Mobiles, ATVs)

Comments: ____________________

Furs

Comments: ____________________

Jewelry

Comments: ____________________

Antiques

Comments: ____________________

Stamps

Comments: ____________________

Coins

Comments: ____________________

Livestock

Comments:

Other

Comments:

PERSONAL ASSETS

Name of Item ________________________

Location of Item ________________________

Appraisal ________________________

Location of Appraisal ________________________

Name of Item ________________________

Location of Item ________________________

Appraisal ________________________

Location of Appraisal ________________________

Name of Item ________________________

Location of Item ________________________

Appraisal ________________________

Location of Appraisal ________________________

Name of Item ________________________

Location of Item ________________________

Appraisal ________________________

Location of Appraisal ________________________

Name of Item ________________________________

Location of Item ________________________________

Appraisal ________________________________

Location of Appraisal ________________________________

Name of Item ________________________________

Location of Item ________________________________

Appraisal ________________________________

Location of Appraisal ________________________________

Name of Item ________________________________

Location of Item ________________________________

Appraisal ________________________________

Location of Appraisal ________________________________

Name of Item ________________________________

Location of Item ________________________________

Appraisal ________________________________

Location of Appraisal ________________________________

Name of Item ________________________________

Location of Item ________________________________

Appraisal ________________________________

Location of Appraisal ________________________________

DISTRIBUTION OF ASSETS*

NOTE: My will is the single best tool for delineating what items of value are to be distributed and to which individual(s). The list below is intended to serve as a backup tool. List here "Item" and name(s) of recipients. I have been as specific as possible. Additional paper has been added as needed on page 233.

How I want my furnishings, jewelry, art, etc. divided among my loved ones :

☛Make every effort to discourage arguments or disputes over personal property from wrecking family relations. Material items never take the place of love for one another.

WHERE TO LOCATE IMPORTANT PAPERS

Credit Cards:

Visa:

Account # ______________________

Location/Comments: ______________________

____

____

MasterCard:

Account # ______________________

Location/Comments: ______________________

____

____

Discover:

Account # ______________________

Location/Comments: ______________________

____

____

American Express:

Account # ______

Other Credit Cards:

Account # ______

Location/Comments: ______

______

______

Account # ______

Location/Comments: ______

______

______

Bank Account Books:

Location/Comments: ______

______

______

Rental Property Payment Books:

Location/Comments: ______

______

______

Other Financial Records:

Location/Comments: ____________________

IMPORTANT KEYS:

Keys to House/Apartment:

Location/Comments: ____________________

Keys to Car(s):

Location/Comments: ____________________

Keys to Safety Deposit Box:

Location/Comments: ____________________

Keys to Office:

Location/Comments: ____________________

Other Important Keys:

Location/Comments: ____________________

WILLS

Two people with copies of my will:

Name ______________________________

Address ______________________________

____

____

Cell Phone # ______________________________

Phone # ______________________________

Name ______________________________

Address ______________________________

____

____

Cell Phone # ______________________________

Phone # ______________________________

POWERS OF ATTORNEY

Two people with Powers of Attorney:

Name ______________________________

Address ______________________________

____

____

Cell Phone # ______________________________

Phone # ______________________________

Name ______________________________

Address ______________________________

____

____

Cell Phone # ______________________________

Phone # ______________________________

BIRTH CERTIFICATE & PASSPORT

BIRTH CERTIFICATE:

Two people with copies of my birth certificate:

Name ______________________

Address ______________________

____

Phone # ______________________

Name ______________________

Address ______________________

____

Phone # ______________________

PASSPORT

Location ______________________

ID# ______________________

Where Issued ______________________

Date Issued ______________________

Expiration Date ______________________

MY MONTHLY BILLS AND OBLIGATIONS*

Name	$Total	Contact Phone#
Mortgage		
Homeowners Dues		
Maintenance		
Utilities		
Gas		
Water		
Monthly		
Electric		
Telephone		
Cable		
Car Payment		
Insurance Premiums		
Regular Health-related		
Other		

*Make copy, post on refrigerator and keep it current.

DEBTS OWED

Type: ____

Name to be paid: ________________________________

Address: ______________________________________

Phone # _______________________________________

Type: ____

Name to be paid: ________________________________

Address: ______________________________________

Phone # _______________________________________

Type: ____

Name to be paid: ________________________________

Address: ______________________________________

Phone # _______________________________________

Type: ____

Name to be paid: ________________________________

Address: ______________________________________

Phone # _______________________________________

IMPORTANT E-MAIL ADDRESSES

Name	E-Mail Address	Reason to Contact

*Keep this list current and perhaps post a copy on your refrigerator. It could prove very helpful.

IMPORTANT HOUSEHOLD INFORMATION & CONTACTS

Garage Door Opener Combination: ______________________

____

Newspaper Delivery Contact: ______________________

Garbage Collection Days: ______________________

Location of Fusebox: ______________________

____

Alarm System

Contact: ______________________

Address: ______________________

Phone # ______________________

Arming Code: ______________________

Disarming Code: ______________________

Location of Water Shut-off: ______________________

Electric Company:

Name ____________________

Phone ____________________

Gas Company:

Name ____________________

Phone ____________________

Plumber:

Name ____________________

Phone ____________________

Electrician:

Name ____________________

Phone ____________________

Lawn Maintenance Person:

Name ____________________

Phone ____________________

Pool Maintenance Person:

Name ____________________

Phone ____________________

Snow Removal:

Name ____________________

Phone ____________________

Heading and Air Conditioning Company:

Name ______________________________

Phone ______________________________

Pest Control:

Name ______________________________

Phone ______________________________

Computer Repair:

Name ______________________________

Phone ______________________________

Auto Repair:

Name ______________________________

Phone ______________________________

Additional Information:

PART III

Personal History

History is an important aspect of every individual's life. Every experience we've had adds to making each of us historic figures in our own right. Some features of our past are significant enough to be included for the education of our future caregivers. Please take the time to provide those individuals with all the historic insight into you, as you would care to share. It may prove very important.

MY CHART OF DECENDANTS

Mother *Father*

Their Children

(me)

married

My Children

My Grandchildren

My Birth:

PERSONAL INFORMATION

Last Name:

First Name:

Middle Name:

Nickname:

Named After:

Birth Date:

Location of BIRTH CERTIFICATE:

Current Address:

Current Telephone Number:

Cell Phone Number:

E-mail Address:

Marriage

Location:

Date:

Location of MARRIAGE CERTIFICATE:

Previous Spouse (If Applicable):

Name:

Address:

Notes:

SPOUSE'S INFORMATION

Last Name:

First Name:

Middle Name:

Nickname:

Named After:

Birth Date:

Location of BIRTH CERTIFICATE:

Current Address:

Current Telephone Number:

Cell Phone Number:

E-mail Address:

Previous Spouse (If Applicable):

Name:

Address:

Notes:

CHILDREN

Full Name:

Date of Birth:

Birthplace:

Current Address:

Current Telephone Number:

Cell Phone Number:

E-mail Address:

Additional Information:

CHILDREN

Full Name:

Date of Birth:

Birthplace:

Current Address:

Current Telephone Number:

Cell Phone Number:

E-mail Address:

Additional Information:

CHILDREN

Full Name: ______

Date of Birth: ______

Birthplace: ______

Current Address: ______

______

______

Current Telephone Number: ______

Cell Phone Number: ______

E-mail Address: ______

Additional Information:

______

______

______

______

______

______

______

______

CHILDREN

Full Name:

Date of Birth:

Birthplace:

Current Address:

Current Telephone Number:

Cell Phone Number:

E-mail Address:

Additional Information:

CHILDREN

Full Name:

Date of Birth:

Birthplace:

Current Address:

Current Telephone Number:

Cell Phone Number:

E-mail Address:

Additional Information:

CHILDREN

Full Name:

Date of Birth:

Birthplace:

Current Address:

Current Telephone Number:

Cell Phone Number:

E-mail Address:

Additional Information:

PARENTS — MOTHER

Maiden Name: ____________________

First Name: ____________________

Middle Name: ____________________

Birth Date: ____________________

Birthplace: ____________________

Current Address: ____________________

____

Current Telephone Number: ____________________

Cell Phone Number: ____________________

E-mail Address: ____________________

Death Date: ____________________

Cause of Death: ____________________

Place of Burial: ____________________

Location: ____________________

Lot#, Grave #, Marker or Monument info): ____________________

____

PARENTS — FATHER

Maiden Name:

First Name:

Middle Name:

Birth Date:

Birthplace:

Current Address:

Current Telephone Number:

Cell Phone Number:

E-mail Address:

Death Date:

Cause of Death:

Place of Burial:

Location:

Lot#, Grave #, Marker or Monument info):

GRANDPARENTS

My ancestors came from the following countries:

Why and when they moved here:

Paternal Grandmother

Full Name:

Date of Birth:

Birthplace:

Current Address:

Date of Death:

Cause of Death:

Place of Burial:

Location (Lot #, Grave #, Marker or Monument info):

Fraternal Grandmother

Full Name:

Date of Birth:

Birthplace:

Current Address:

Date of Death:

Cause of Death:

Place of Burial:

Location (Lot #, Grave #, Marker or Monument info):

Paternal Grandfather

Full Name:

Date of Birth:

Birthplace:

Current Address:

Date of Death:

Cause of Death:

Place of Burial:

Location (Lot #, Grave #, Marker or Monument info):

Fraternal Grandfather

Full Name:

Date of Birth:

Birthplace:

Current Address:

Date of Death:

Cause of Death:

Place of Burial:

Location (Lot #, Grave #, Marker or Monument info):

FAMILY MEMORIES

What I know of my family's history prior to my birth:

Who most influenced my life (How?):

Advice or philosophy of life I want to pass on to my children and/or grandchildren:

The one thing I did in my life that made me the happiest or most proud — my greatest accomplishment:

The most unique and memorable experiences in my life.

Author's examples:

- Sat in the President's box at the Kennedy Center as guest of President Johnson.
- Lived in Fontainebleau, France.
- Travelled to Hawaii to meet husband on R&R from Vietnam.
- Once sat next to the President of South Korea
- Met so many interesting people when my daughter Robin was co-host of TV's "Doubledare" on Nickelodeon.

EDUCATION

Elementary School

Name:

Location:

Junior High or Middle School

Name:

Location:

High School

Name:

Location:

College/University

Undergraduate:

Location:

Major:

Minor:

Degree Received:

Honors:

Graduate:

Location:

Major:

Degree Received:

Additional Educational Information:

MILITARY HISTORY

- I served from: ________ to: ________ in the:

  ________ Army

  ________ Air Force

  ________ Navy

  ________ Marines

  ________ Merchant Marines

  ________ Coast Guard

  ________ Other Service ____________________

- My rank at discharge was:

  ____

- My discharge date was (day, month, year):

  ____

- My discharge papers are filed (location):

  ____

- I belong to the following veterans' organizations:

  ____

  ____

The most memorable event(s) of my time in the military:

CAREER

Company Name:

Location: ____

Job Title/Description: ____

Years Employed: ____

Company Name:

Location: ____

Job Title/Description: ____

Years Employed: ____

Company Name:

Location: ____

Job Title/Description: ____

Years Employed: ____

Notes:

THROUGH THE YEARS

It is important to fill in this section. If someday , you are diagnosed with Alzheimer's, your loved ones will have points of reference when speaking with you. (Alzheimer's patients remember the past more often than the present.)

IN MY TEENS:

I lived in:

- City / State ______

High School and year of graduation:

- Name / Date ______

My favorite date was (his/her name):

- ______

My favorite thing to do on a date was:

- ______

For fun, my friends and I would:

My interests and hobbies were:

Additional information:

IN MY 20'S

I lived in:

- City / State ______________________

I worked at:

- Company/Job ______________________

I married: ______________________

on ______________________. (month/day/year)

My children's names are:

- ______________ /DOB ______________
- ______________ /DOB ______________
- ______________ /DOB ______________
- ______________ /DOB ______________

My friends included:

- ______________________
- ______________________
- ______________________
- ______________________
- ______________________

For fun, my friends and I would:

My interests and hobbies were:

Additional information:

IN MY 30'S

I lived in:

- City / State ______

I worked at:

- Company/Job ______

I married: ______

on ______. (month/day/year)

My children's names are:

- ______ /DOB ______
- ______ /DOB ______
- ______ /DOB ______
- ______ /DOB ______

My friends included:

- ______
- ______
- ______
- ______
- ______

For fun, my friends and I would:

My interests and hobbies were:

Additional information:

IN MY 40'S

I lived in:

City / State ______

I worked at:

Company/Job ______

My grandchildren's names are:

______ /DOB ______

______ /DOB ______

______ /DOB ______

______ /DOB ______

My friends included:

______

______

______

______

______

______

______

______

For fun, my friends and I would:

My interests and hobbies were:

Additional information:

IN MY 50'S

I lived in:

- City / State ______

I worked at:

- Company/Job ______

My grandchildren's names are:

- ______ /DOB ______
- ______ /DOB ______
- ______ /DOB ______
- ______ /DOB ______

My friends included:

- ______
- ______
- ______
- ______
- ______
- ______
- ______
- ______

For fun, my friends and I would:

My interests and hobbies were:

Additional information:

IN MY 60'S

I lived in:

- City / State ______

I worked at:

- Company/Job ______

My grandchildren's names are:

- ______ /DOB ______
- ______ /DOB ______
- ______ /DOB ______
- ______ /DOB ______

My friends included:

- ______
- ______
- ______
- ______
- ______
- ______
- ______
- ______

For fun, my friends and I would:

My interests and hobbies were:

Additional information:

IN MY 70'S

I lived in:

- City / State ____________________

I worked at:

- Company/Job ____________________

My grandchildren's names(Great grandchildren if there are any):

- ________________ /DOB ________________
- ________________ /DOB ________________
- ________________ /DOB ________________
- ________________ /DOB ________________

My friends included:

- ________________________________
- ________________________________
- ________________________________
- ________________________________
- ________________________________
- ________________________________
- ________________________________
- ________________________________

For fun, my friends and I would:

My interests and hobbies were:

Additional information:

IN MY 80'S

I lived in:

- City / State ______

My grandchildren's names(Great grandchildren if there are any):

- ______ /DOB ______
- ______ /DOB ______
- ______ /DOB ______
- ______ /DOB ______
- ______ /DOB ______
- ______ /DOB ______

My friends included:

- ______
- ______
- ______
- ______
- ______
- ______
- ______
- ______

For fun, my friends and I would:

My interests and hobbies were:

Additional information:

MY POST-80'S YEARS

Things I want remembered about these days in my life:

TRADITIONAL FAMILY HOLIDAYS

Holiday ______________________________

Family Tradition Observed ______________________________

____

____

____

Holiday ______________________________

Family Tradition Observed ______________________________

____

____

____

NOTE: For many people, Thanksgiving and Halloween are typical holidays that are observed. However, since there are many holidays throughout any given year, and considering that we all celebrate different ones in our own family structure (e.g., Christmas, Easter, Hanukkah, Ramadan, Kwanzaa), please fill in the ones you honor.

Holiday

Family Tradition Observed

Holiday

Family Tradition Observed

Holiday

Family Tradition Observed

My favorite holiday:

Why this holiday has always been so special:

What I love to do on my favorite holiday:

Holiday vacation(s) I have enjoyed the most (such as a visit to the seashore, to the mountains, taking a cruise, etc.):

PART VI

Appendices

INTERNET RESOURCES

These resources are recommended for your consideration and review. As you age, it is your personal responsibility to stay educated and on top of key issues that are or will be impacting your life. This list is only as good or as valuable as you make it. Be sure to add new sites to this list as you uncover them.

Please keep one thing in mind: You are taking steps to address issues in your own future and speak to those caregivers that will be working with you at that time. There are very few resources that currently address "future" issues in caregiving. You may have to be creative.

Alzheimer's Association
www.ahaf.org/alzheimers/livingwith/caregiving.html

AARP
General Information: *www.aarp.org*
Independent Living: *www.aarp.org/family/caregiving*
Taxes: *www.aarp.org/taxaide*
Public Benefits Outreach Program: *www.aarp.org/money/lowincomehelp*

AMA (American Medical Association)
www.ama-assn.org

AMA Doctor Finder
http://webapps.ama-assn.org/doctorfinder/home.html

CancerCare
www.cancercare.org

Cancer Caregiving
www.cancercaregiving.com

Cancer.net (American Society of Clinical Oncology)
Home: *www.asco.org*
Caregiving: *www.asco.org/patient/Coping/Caregiving*

Caregiver's Home Companion
www.caregivershome.com

Caregiving.com
www.caregiving.com

Caring.com
www.caring.com

Caring Connections
www.caringinfo.org/caringforsomeone

Compare Hospitals

www.hospitalcompare.hhs.gov

Complaints

www.healthfinder.gov/scripts/SearchContext.asp?topic=14309&Branch=3

Elder Care Locator

www.eldercare.gov/Eldercare/Public/Home.asp

Family Caregiving 101

www.familycaregiving101.org

Family Caregiver Alliance

www.caregiver.org/caregiver/jsp/home.jsp

Find a Facility

www.healthfinder.gov/scripts/Topics.asp?context=8&keyword=147&Branch=3

Healthcare Quality

www.ahrq.gov/consumer/guidetoq

Healthy Aging (Centers for Disease Control)

www.cdc.gov/aging/caregiving/index.htm

Heart of Caregiving

www.americanheart.org/presenter.jhtml?identifier=3039829

Health Insurance

www.healthinsuranceinfo.net

HIPAA

www.healthfinder.gov/scripts/SearchContext.asp?topic=5706&Branch=3

Hospice

www.hospicenet.org

www.nhpco.org/custom/directory/main.cfm

Long-Term Care

www.longtermcareliving.com

Lotsa Helping Hands

www.lotsahelpinghands.com

Managed Care

www.pohly.com/terms.html

Mayo Clinic

www.mayoclinic.com

www.mayoclinic.com/health/alzheimers/AZ00013

Medicare

Home: *www.medicare.gov*

Medicare Health Plans:
www.medicare.gov/MPPF/Include/DataSection/Questions/Welcome.asp

Medication Errors

www.fda.gov/cder/drug/mederrors/default.htm

MedicineNet.com

www.medicinenet.com/caregiving/article.htm

MedlinePlus (National Institutes of Health)

www.nlm.nih.gov/medlineplus/caregivers.html

My Care Community

www.mycarecommunity.org

National Alliance for Caregivers

www.caregiving.org

National Association for Home Care and Hospice

www.nahc.org

National Caregiving Association

www.caregivingfoundation.org

National Family Caregivers Association

www.nfcacares.org

National Family Caregiver Support Program (Dept. of Health and Human Services)

www.aoa.gov/prof/aoaprog/caregiver/careprof/progguidance/resources/caregiving_terms.aspx

Quality Care Connections
(Rosalynn Carter Institute for Caregiving and Johnson & Johnson)

www.qualitycareconnections.org/QCC/Welcome.html

Patient Records Confidentiality

www.ama-assn.org/ama/pub/category/4610.html

Power of Attorney

http://www.uslegalforms.com/poweratty.htm

Prevention Magazine

www.prevention.com/cda/homepage.do

Privacy

www.ama-assn.org/ama/pub/category/4610.html

Privacy Myths

www.myphr.com/rights/common_myths.asp

Rosalynn Carter Institute for Caregiving

www.rosalynncarter.org/

www.qualitycareconnections.org/QCC/Welcome.html

Social Security

Strength for Caring (sponsored by Johnson & Johnson)

www.strengthforcaring.com/

Suite 101

www.suite101.com/welcome.cfm/elderly_caregiving

Support Groups

www.healthfinder.gov/scripts/SearchContext.asp?topic=833&Branch=3

The Center for Volunteer Caregiving

www.volunteercaregiving.org

Third Age

www.thirdage.com/caregiving

Veterans Benefits

Military Records Request: *http://www.archives.gov*
National Cemetery Administration: *http://www.cem.va.gov/*
VA Facility Directory: *http://www1.va.gov*
Veterans Health Administration: *http://www.appc1.va.gov*
Veterans Benefits Administration: *http://www.va.gov/*
Federal Benefits For Veterans: *http://www1.va.gov/opa/vadocs/Fedben.pdf*

Understand Your Medications

www.usp.org/pdf/EN/patientSafety/justAskDozenQs.pdf

Visiting Nurse Association

http://vnaa.org/vnaa/gen/HTML~Home.aspx

Finding a visiting nurse in your area:
http://www.vnaa.org/vnaa/Searches/findvna.aspx

WebMD

www.webmd.com/healthy-aging/caregiving-insights/default.htm

Well Spouse Association

www.wellspouse.org

Wiser Women Institute for a Secure Retirement

www.wiserwomen.org/portal/index.php?option=com_frontpage&Itemid=1

WORDS & PHRASES TO KEEP HANDY

On the following pages, you have been provided with the major terms that are being used in newspapers, magazines, on TV and the radio when discussing issues impacting Americans at the time of publication. The author and publisher believe these are important words and phrases with which you should become familiar and conversant. Should you find that some of these words become very much a part of your life, you might improve your understanding by reading up on them by visiting the library near your home and by making use of the wide array of information available on the Internet.

***NOTE:** DC Press does not offer legal advice. Prior to attempting to utilize any form presented in this book or when making an important decision effecting your future healthcare or finances, seek the advise of a legal, accounting, and/or medical professionals.

A

Acute Care

Special care that is provided typically for a brief period of time to treat a certain illness or condition. This type of care often includes short-term hospital stays, doctor's visits, surgery, and X-rays.

Adult Care Home

A residence that offers services of a housing and personal care nature for 3 up to 16 residents. The owner or manager usually provides services such as meals, supervision, and transportation. Can also be known as a board and care home or group home.

Advance Directive for Health Care

Legal document, such as a living will, a durable power of attorney for healthcare, or both), prepared ahead of time and signed by a living and competent person in order to provide guidance for medical and health-care decisions (including the termination of life support and organ donation) in the event that he or she becomes incompetent to make such decisions.

Alzheimer's Disease

A progressive, irreversible disease of unknown cause that is the most common form of dementia, marked by the loss of cognitive ability (due to degeneration of the brain cells and serve loss of memory). It usually starts in late middle age or in old age as a loss of memory of recent events, which spreads to memories for more distant events. It progresses on average over the course of five to ten or fifteen years to a profound intellectual decline characterized by dementia and personal helplessness.

Assisted Living Facility

Often licensed and known as residential care facilities or rest homes, a residence that combines housing, supportive services, personalized assistance and healthcare designed to meet the individual's needs on a daily basis emphasizing residents' privacy and choice. These needs may include bathing, dressing, balancing a checkbook, medication reminders, and/or Housework for example. In many assisted living facilities, 24-hour supportive services are available to meet the planned and unplanned needs of the residents. These settings in which services are delivered may include self-contained apartment units or single or shared room units with private or area baths. Assisted Living Facilities can be similar to a Board and Care Home, but are typically larger.

Assistive Devices

A range of products designed to help elders or people with disabilities lead more independent lives. Examples include walking aids, motorized wheelchairs, lifts, raised/elevated toilet seats, bathtub seats, ramps, and handrails for example. In some cases, modifications to the living facility are required in order to properly utilize the devices. Also known as Architectural Adaptations, these are structural fabrications or remodeling in the home, work site, or other areas (including for example ramps, lifts, lighting, kitchen remodeling, bathroom adaptations) that remove or reduce physical barriers for an individual with a disability.

B

Beneficiary

A person or entity (perhaps a charity or estate) that receives a benefit or proceeds from something, a person or entity named or otherwise entitled to receive the proceeds (principal or income or both) from a will, trust, insurance policy, retirement plan, annuity or other contract. An individual covered by Medicare is also called a beneficiary.

Benefit Trigger

Before benefits are paid, certain benefit triggers and other conditions must be met. A benefit trigger is usually met by measuring a person's ability to do one or more activities of daily living (ADLs), such as bathing or dressing, or by testing the person's cognitive abilities. Also, it is a condition that must exist in order for an insurance company to pay benefits under a long-term care insurance policy. Benefits are triggered for nursing home care, assisted living, or home care when a person can't do two of the ADLs listed in the policy, or when a person has an obvious cognitive impairment like Alzheimer's and has met other conditions in the policy. Tax-qualified policies use a list of six ADLs: Bathing, Dressing, Transferring, Eating, Toileting, and Continence

Non-tax qualified policies use seven ADLs, adding ambulating (walking) to the list.

Benefits

A monetary sum or payment made or an entitlement available in accordance with an insurance policy or a public assistance program, or to someone else, such as a health care provider, to whom the insured person has assigned the benefits.

Board and Care Home

A Board and Care Home usually offers seniors supervision and some personal care (such as meals and transportation), but few onsite medical services. A small number of residents live (between 3 and 16) in a group home, sometimes in a refurbished single-family home. A Board and Care Home can be the same as an Assisted Living Facility, but on a smaller scale.

C

Care/Case Management

Care management is a coordinated care function (single point of entry)

incorporating case finding, assessment, care planning, negotiation, care plan implementation, monitoring, and advocacy to assist clients and their families with complex needs in obtaining appropriate services. This program (operated privately or through social service agencies or public programs) locates, mobilizes and manages a variety of home care and other services needed by a frail elderly person at risk of nursing home placement. An assessment is performed to identify needs, and appropriate services are secured to enable the individual to remain at home. Case managers assist in gaining access to needed services for those persons eligible. They monitor the provision of these services as well as initiate and oversee the assessment and reassessment of an individual's level and plan of care.

Care Manager

A health care professional, typically a nurse or social worker, who arranges, monitors, or coordinates long-term care services. A care manager may also assess a patient's needs and develop a plan of care, subject to approval by the patient's physician. They may also be referred to as a care coordinator or case manager.

Chore Services

In short, they are assistance with chores such as home repairs, yard work, and heavy housecleaning. They are non-continuous household maintenance tasks intended to increase the safety of the individual(s) in their residence(s). Typically these tasks are limited to the following: replacing light bulbs, fuses, electric plugs and frayed cords, door locks, window catches, water pipes, faucets and/or washers. They can include installation and repair of safety equipment, screens and storm windows, weather stripping around doors, window shades and curtain rods. Furniture repair, the cleaning of appliances, rugs, basements and attics to remove potential hazards are included. As are washing walls and windows, scrubbing floors, pest control, mowing grass and raking leaves, clearing ice, snow, and leaves from sidewalks, driveways, and step, and trimming overhanging branches.

Chronically Ill Individual

A chronically ill individual, as defined by the federal government, is someone who has been certified (at least in the past twelve months) by a licensed health care practitioner as — (1) Being unable to perform, without substantial assistance from another individual, at least two daily living activities (eating, toileting, transferring, bathing, dressing, and continence) for at least 90 days due to a loss of functional capacity or (2) Requiring substantial supervision to protect the individual from threats to health and safety due to severe cognitive impairment.

Chronic Illness or Condition

There are two types of illnesses: acute and chronic. Acute illnesses (like a cold or the flu) are usually over relatively quickly. Chronic illnesses, though, are long-lasting health conditions (the word "chronic" comes from the Greek word chronos, meaning time). An illness or other condition with one or more of the following characteristics: permanency, residual disability, requires rehabilitation training, or requires a long period of supervision, observation, or care. Typically, it is a disease or condition that lasts over a long period of time and cannot be cured; it is often associated with disability.

Codicil

A supplement, appendix, or legal change to a will.

Congregate Housing

Congregate (or supported) housing is a group housing option (such as individual apartments) for the elderly and disabled, with private living quarters and common dining and social areas with additional safety measures such as emergency call buttons. Support services vary, but usually include meals, housekeeping and activities. People living in a congregate housing facility require little or no personal care assistance.

Continuing Care Retirement Community (CCRC)

A are privately owned privately owned retirement community for people who cannot or who prefer not to maintain an independent household because they need some kind of long-term assistance or medical care that offer a broad range of services and degrees or levels of care based on individual needs. Also known as life care, these communities can range from full-time care in nursing homes to assisted living to independent living situations. It is not unusual for continuing care retirement communities (CCRCs) to be expensive and entry fees or payments required prior to acceptance along with continuing monthly fees.

Custodial Care

Room and board in a nursing home where assistance with activities of daily living is provided such as bathing, dressing, eating, and other non-medical care that most people do themselves. Medicare does not pay for custodial care. Medicaid provides the majority of reimbursement for custodial care, although very little. It is important to note that it is typical that individuals without professional training may provide this type of care.

D

Dementia

Dementia is a progressive brain dysfunction that leads to a gradually increasing restriction of daily activities, the deterioration of intellectual abilities such as vocabulary, abstract thinking, judgment, memory loss, and physical coordination. Alzheimer's disease is the best-known type of dementia. Dementia seriously affects patients as well as those around them. Most patients eventually require care in the long-term. Some degenerative diseases, vascular diseases or stroke, metabolic disorders, drugs and alcohol, and psychiatric disorders can cause dementia.

Depression

Depression is an illness that affects both mind and body—one that can make it difficult to handle everyday life. It is one of the most undiagnosed conditions among seniors. Research has linked depression to an imbalance in two of the naturally occurring chemicals in the brain and body, serotonin and norepinephrine. These chemicals help regulate how your body perceives thoughts and feelings—including pain. While people with a family history of depression may be more prone to the disease, anyone can become depressed. Sometimes the triggers are external—for example, relationship troubles or financial problems; at other times the disease can be brought about by physical illness or hormonal shifts. Depression can also occur without any identifiable trigger at all. Symptoms can include a persistent sad, anxious or "empty" mood, loss of interest or pleasure in activities once enjoyed and difficulty sleeping.

Discharge Planner

A health care professional or social worker who assists hospital patients and their families in transitioning from the hospital to another level of care such as a rehabilitation center, rehabilitation in a skilled nursing facility, home health care in the patient's home, or long-term care in a nursing home.

Do Not Resuscitate Order

A code or order usually appearing in a patient's medical record indicating that in the event the heart and/or breathing stops, no intervention be undertaken by staff. Death occurs undisturbed. This does not mean that the individual does not receive care. Continuing care is provided as it would to any individual (medications for pain, antibiotics, etc.) except as stated above.

Durable Medical Equipment

Known as DME (also known as Home Medical Equipment), this is equipment that: can be used over and over again, is ordinarily used for medical purposes, and is generally not useful to a person who isn't sick, injured or disabled. Initially, it is medical equipment ordered by a doctor who writes a prescription for it for use in the home. Equipment includes canes, crutches, walkers, hospital beds, wheelchairs, lifts, and prosthetics used at home. DME may be covered by Medicaid and in part by Medicare or private insurance.

E

Elder Care

A relatively new and growing area of health care that is concerned with providing medical and other services for the rapidly growing, aging population —typically persons 65 and older. It consists of a wide range of services provided at home, throughout the community, and in residential care facilities, which includes assisted living facilities and nursing homes. It can include such health-related services as rehabilitative therapies, skilled nursing, and palliative care. It also includes supervision and a wide range of supportive personal care and social services. Elder care is usually provided over an extended period of time to individuals needing the assistance of others to perform normal daily living activities due to cognitive impairment or loss of muscular strength or control. Typically Medicare does not cover the majority of elder care because it is viewed as custodial care.

Estate

The whole of one's possessions, especially all the property and debts left by one at death.

Executor

The person or institution appointed by a court or testator to execute his will, or to see its provisions carried into effect, after his decease.

F

Fiduciary

A person, such as a trustee or guardian, who holds assets of another person or beneficiary, often with the legal authority and duty to make decisions regarding financial matters on behalf of the other party. It is illegal for a fiduciary to misappropriate money for personal gain.

Family Medical Leave Act

Known as FMLA, the Federal law that requires any firm with over 50 employees to grant an eligible employee up to a total of 12 work weeks of unpaid leave during any 12-month period to care for a family member with a serious health condition —such as a senior. The employer must maintain an employee's group health insurance benefits while taking FMLA leave and must reinstate the employee in the same job upon returning from FMLA leave.

G

Geriatric Care Manager

Geriatric Care Managers provide a variety of services for seniors and caregivers including assessment, planning and management of home and health care for seniors. Also known as senior care managers, a geriatric care manager generally conducts an interview and provides a home assessment before creating a senior care plan with recommendations.

Geriatrician

A geriatrician is a doctor who specializes in care for people 65 and older, caring for the special and changing needs of seniors. Geriatricians approach each patient's needs individually, and possess the knowledge and expertise needed to accommodate complex medical and social concerns.

Guardian

One who is legally responsible (appointed by a court) for the care and management of the person or property of an individual who is unable to take care of himself or herself.

H

Health Maintenance Organization

Known as an HMO, group insurance that entitles members to services of participating hospitals, clinics and physicians. For those aged 65 and older, a type of Medicare managed care plan where a group of doctors, hospitals and other health care providers agree to give health care to Medicare beneficiaries for a pre-established amount of money from Medicare every month. Typically members must get all of their care from the providers who participate in the plan. Use of providers outside the HMO, will require payment out of pocket for services.

Heir

Someone who inherits assets from an estate of another person who has died. The heir does not have to pay income tax or estate tax on the value of the inheritance received.

Home Care

Caring for an aging or impaired person in their home by providing homemaking, meal preparation, shopping, transportation and assistance with activities of daily living.

Home Care Aides

Individuals who provide non-medical assistance to impaired individuals in their homes.

Home Health Agency (HHA)

Also known as an HHA, this is a public or private operation providing home health services which are supervised by a licensed health professional in the patient's home either directly or through arrangements with other organizations.

Home Health Care

Generally, home health services are initiated when an individual is no longer able to care for him or herself due to serious changes in their health. It is not unusual for a doctor, nurse, hospital discharge planner or case manager to suggest that professional help in the home, as an alternative to hospitalization or a nursing home, to assist with health care needs on a round-the-clock basis —although home health care services are usually provided on a visit basis rather than an hourly basis. Readmission to a hospital can often be prevented or delayed. Most services must be ordered by a physician, and must be medically necessary to maintain or improve your health condition, in order to be covered by health insurance. Home health care services are usually provided on a visit basis rather than an hourly basis.

Homebound

An individual is understood to be homebound if absences from the home are infrequent or of relatively short duration, or are attributable to the need to receive medical treatment. Leaving home to receive medical treatment includes going to adult day care so long as the individual receives therapeutic, psychosocial or medical treatment from a licensed or state-certified adult day-care facility. Any absence for a religious service is considered an absence of short duration and doesn't negate the homebound status.

Hospice and Hospice Care

This is a program providing palliative care that improves the quality of life of patients facing terminal illness (end-of-life) and their families. The prevention and relief of suffering by means of early identification and impeccable assessment and treatment of pain and other problems, physical, psychosocial and spiritual is all part of the program. Hospices 1) provide relief from pain and other distressing symptoms, 2) affirm life and regard dying as a normal process, 3) neither hasten or postpone death intentionally, 4) integrate both psychological and spiritual aspects of patient care, 5) offer a support system to help patients live as actively as possible until death, 6) offer a support system to help the family cope during the patient's illness and through bereavement, 7) use a team approach to address the needs of patients and their families, including bereavement counseling, when needed, (8) are designed to enhance quality of life, and may also positively influence the course of an illness, and 9) are applicable early in the course of illness, in conjunction with other therapies that are intended to prolong life, such as radiation or chemotherapy, and includes those investigations needed to better understand and manage distressing clinical complications. Hospice care can be provided at home, in a facility with a homelike setting, a hospital or a nursing home. The care includes physical care, counseling and support services, but does not attempt to cure any illness.

I

Independent Living Facility

A type of living arrangement in which personal care services such as meals, housekeeping, transportation, and assistance with activities of daily living are available as needed to people who still live on their own in a residential facility. In most cases, the "assisted living" residents pay a regular monthly rent. They typically pay additional fees for the services they get.

Instrumental Activities of Daily Living

Instrumental activities of daily living (also known as IADLs) are activities related to independent living (without the assistance or substantial supervision of another person) and include for example grocery shopping and preparing meals, managing money, shopping for groceries or personal items, performing light or heavy housework, doing laundry, using a telephone, paying bills, and taking daily medications. Most long-term care insurance policies will not pay benefits for the loss of ability to perform IADLs.

Intermediate Care

Needed for people in stable condition who require daily care, but not round-the clock nursing supervision. Typically ordered by a doctor and supervised by registered nurses. Intermediate care is less specialized than skilled nursing care and it usually involves more personal care.

Intermediate care is generally needed for a long period of time.

Intermediate Care Facility

Nursing homes most frequently come to mind when people envision what is in reality an intermediate care facility (also known as an ICF). Recognized under the Medicaid program, they provides health-related care and services to individuals who do not require acute or skilled nursing care, but who, because of their mental or physical condition, require care and services above the level of room and board available only through facility placement. These facilities often have more mobile, less acutely ill residents than a skilled nursing facility, which provides sophisticated medical care to people with acute medical needs. An ICF is staffed by a team of nurses under the supervision of an attending physician. Much of the care provided in an ICF--often called "custodial" or "maintenance care" and provided in large part by nurses' aides--is personal care like help with bathing, dressing, and eating. An ICF is often set up as a wing of a skilled nursing facility. Specific requirements for ICF's vary by state. Institutions for care of the mentally retarded or people with related conditions (ICF/MR) are also included. The distinction between "health-related care and services" and "room and board" is important since ICF's are subject to different regulations and coverage requirements than institutions that do not provide health-related care and services.

J

Joint Tenancy with Right of Survivorship

Ownership of property by two or more people in which the survivors automatically gain ownership of a decedent's interest. Upon the death of any joint tenant, his or her ownership interest automatically passes to the surviving joint tenant.

L

Level of Care

Known as LOC, an assessment of the type of care necessary to meet the individual needs of the client and their eligibility for programs and services. The assessment takes into consideration the client's needs in all aspects of development, level of functioning (levels include: protective, intermediate, and skilled), and potential to benefit from a particular program.

Life Care Plan

Specific plan developed by a professional known as a Life Care Planner. An important tool in the future of a catastrophically injured person (such as on the job, in a serious accident, through medical malpractice). The Life Care Planner summarizes the medical, educational, vocational, psychosocial, and daily living needs of the individual who can function indefinitely only with professional assistance. The Life Care Planner projects the long-term costs of care, and establishes rehabilitative goals while coordinating future care providers in order to best assure a continued recovery.

Living Trust

A trust created for and individual (the trustor) and administered by another party during the trustor's lifetime. The living trust may be formed because the trustor is either incapable of managing or unwilling to manage his or her assets. The trust can be revocable or irrevocable, depending upon the trustor's wishes. It avoids probate and assests are distributed typically faster than through a will. Also called an inter vivos trust.

Living Will

A legal document (a will) in which the signer requests not to be kept alive by medical life-support systems in the event of a terminal illness or incapacity..

Long-Term Care

Term used to represent a range of services that address the health, social, and personal care needs of individuals delivered over a long period of time to persons who have never developed or have lost some capacity for self care.

Long-Term Care Insurance

An insurance policy that provides benefits for the chronically ill or disabled over a long period of time that helps pay for some long-term medical and non-medical care, such as help with activities of daily living. Medicare typically does not pay for long-term care.

M

Managed Care

A system of health care that combines delivery and payment; and influences utilization of services, by employing management techniques designed to promote the delivery of cost-effective health care. Organizations created included MNOs, PPOs, and PSOs. Members pay a pre-established monthly amount for care to be provided regardless of the amount required.

Medicaid

Health care for the aged administered by the federal and state governments. A program dependent upon low level of income and assets relative to high level of medical/health care bills. Coverage and eligibility requirements vary from state-to-state. The primary payer of nursing home care. Some states offer home and community-based long-term care services for eligible individuals through their individual programs and are at the option of those states and are not mandated by federal law.

Medicare

A program under the U.S. Social Security Administration that reimburses hospitals and physicians for medical care provided to qualifying people over 65 years and to some younger people who are very ill or disabled. Benefits for nursing home and short-term home health services are limited and are generally available only to people while they are recovering from an acute illness. Coverage is restricted to medical care, and does not include prescription drugs or custodial care at home or in nursing homes.

Medicare HMOs

An HMO (Health Maintenance Organization) is a health plan that is also involved in how an individual's health care is delivered. Managed care refers to health plans coordinating one's health care with the individual and the providers that participate in the health plan. HMOs are the most common type of managed care. A Medicare HMO is an HMO that has contracted with the federal government under the Medicare+ Choice program to provide health benefits to individuals eligible for Medicare that choose to enroll in the HMO, instead of receiving their benefits and care through the traditional fee for service Medicare program. Members pay their regular monthly premiums to Medicare, and Medicare pays the HMO a fixed sum of money each month to provide Medicare benefits (such as hospitalization, doctor's visits, etc.). Medicare HMOs may provide extra benefits over and above regular Medicare benefits (such as prescription drug coverage, eyeglasses, etc.). Members do not pay Medicare deductibles and co-payments; however, the HMO may require them to pay an additional monthly premium and co-payments for some services. If members use providers outside the HMO's network, they pay the entire bill themselves unless the plan has a point of service option.

Medicare Supplement Insurance

Medicare supplement insurance helps pay expenses not covered by original Medicare (often referred to as MedSupp), such as deductibles and coinsurance and was designed to fill in the gaps left by Medicare.. However, non-covered charges will be the insured's responsibility. Policies that meet the definition of Medicare supplement insurance are clearly labeled, usually on the policy's front cover. May pay for some limited long-term care expenses, depending on the benefits package purchased. Also called Medigap.

Medical Power of Attorney

An advance directive with written instructions that appoint someone to make decisions about an individual's medical care.

N

Nursing Home

Filling a special niche in health care, a private facility that provides living quarters and care for the elderly or the chronically ill who do not need the intensive, acute care of a hospital but for whom remaining home is no longer appropriate. Licensed by the state, it offers residents personal care as well as skilled nursing care on a 24-hour basis. Nursing homes are capable of caring for individuals with a wide range of medical conditions. Provides nursing care, personal care, room and board, supervision, medication, therapies and rehabilitation.

Nursing homes come in different sizes and with different names. They may also be known as: health centers, havens or manors, homes for the aged, nursing homes or centers, care centers, continuing care centers, living centers, or convalescent centers.

Nurse Practitioner

Known as an NP, a registered nurse working in an expanded nursing role, usually with a focus on meeting primary health care needs. They conduct physical examinations, interpret laboratory results, select plans of treatment, identify medication requirements, and perform certain medical management activities for selected health conditions. Some specialize in geriatric care.

O

Ombudsman

A representative who investigates complaints and mediates fair settlements for a public agency or a private nonprofit, especially between aggrieved parties such as older consumers who reside in long-term care facilities and the facility, institution or organization.

Outpatient

A patient who does not reside in or has not been admitted to the hospital where they are being treated and receiving ambulatory care.

P

Personal Emergency Response System

In case of a fall or other medical emergency, An electronic device enables the user to contact assistance 24-hours-a-day simply by pressing a button in the event of an emergency (personal medical issue, a fall, fire, etc.)

Physician Assistant

A specially trained and licensed or otherwise credentialed individual who performs tasks under the direction of a supervising physician which might otherwise be performed by a physician. Usually called a PA.

Plan of Care

A written plan describing what specific services and care needed for an individual's health problem. An individual's plan of care must be prepared or approved by their doctor.

Point-of-Service Plan

A health plan that allows members to choose to receive services from a participating or non-participating network provider, usually with a financial disincentive for going outside the network. More of a product than an organization, POS plans can be offered by HMOs, PPOs, or self-insured employers.

Power of Attorney

A General Power of Attorney is a legal document which gives the person you choose (the agent) the power to manage your assets and financial affairs while you are alive. The simplest and least expensive legal device for authorizing a person to manage the affairs of another. The document must be signed by an individual (the principal) while that person has the required legal capacity to give their agent clear and concise instructions. The appointment may be for a fixed period and can be revoked by the individual at any time providing he or she still has the legal capacity to do so. A power of attorney ceases when the individual dies. The executor named in your will then takes over the responsibilities of your estate.

A Durable Power of Attorney stays valid even if you become unable to handle your own affairs (incapacitated). If you don't specify that you want your power of attorney to be durable, it will automatically end if you later become incapacitated

A Limited Power of Attorney allows the principal to give only specific powers to the agent. The limited power of attorney is used to allow the agent to handle specific matters when the principal is unavailable or unable to do so.

Forms needed for specific states may be found at: *http://www.uslegalforms.com/poweratty.htm.*

Power of Attorney for Health Care

Allows an individual to appoint a person to make medical decisions for them in the event they are unable to do so for themselves. A written legal document in which one person (the principal) appoints another person to make health care decisions on behalf of the principal in the event the principal becomes incapacitated (the document defines incapacitation). This instrument can contain instructions about specific medical treatment that should be applied or withheld. While its purpose remains essentially the same from state-to-state, the name of this document can vary; for example, in Florida it is called a Designation of Health Care Surrogate.

Forms needed for specific states may be found at: *http://www.uslegalforms.com/poweratty.htm.*

Preferred Provider Organization

A type of managed care plan (known as a PPO). Members have a choice of utilizing healthcare providers in the PPO network, or hospitals, doctors and other healthcare professionals outside the plan for an additional cost.

Primary Care Physician

Physician responsible for a person's general or basic health care (known as General Practitioner or Family Doctor). The physician an individual sees first for most health problems. They make sure you get the care needed to stay healthy. They might talk with other more specialized doctors and healthcare providers and make a referral to them. In many Medicare managed care plans, participants must see their primary care doctor before seeing other healthcare providers.

Primary Caregiver

The individual or individuals, usually the spouse or adult child, over the age of eighteen years designated by a qualified patient who has consistently assumed responsibility for the housing, health or safety of that qualified patient on a day-by-day basis. They take responsibility for caring for the physical, psychological and social needs of another individual.

Probate

Proof that a will is valid and that its terms are being carried out. Probate is accomplished by an executor/executrix (if a will exists) who is paid a fee based on the size of the estate that passes through the will. Certain trusts and jointly owned property pass to beneficiaries without being subject to probate and the attendant fee. Executor or a court-appointed administrator (if there is no will), manages and distributes a decedent's property to heirs and/or beneficiaries.

Provider

A person or organization who helps in identifying or preventing or treating illness and/or disability.

These can be any of the following: a properly-licensed doctor, health care professional, hospital, or other health care facility, including a home health agency, that provides health care or related social services.

Provider Sponsored Organization

Similar to an HMO or Medicare HMO except that this managed care organization (known as a PSO) is owned by the providers in that plan and these providers share the financial risk assumed by the organization.

R

Rehabilitation Services

Services designed to improve/restore a person's functioning; includes physical therapy, occupational therapy, and/or speech therapy. May be provided at home or in long-term care facilities. May be covered in part by Medicare. Because rehabilitation services are an optional Medicaid benefit, not all states provide this service.

Residential Care

Room, board and personal care provided in a fashion that falls between the nursing care delivered in skilled and intermediate care facilities and the assistance provided through social services. Typically 24-hour supervision is provided to individuals requiring assistance with daily living activities.

Residential Care Facility

Generic term for group homes, specialized apartment complexes, or other institutions providing care services (room, board and personal care) for residents. The term is used to refer to a range of residential care options including assisted living facilities, board and care homes and skilled nursing facilities providing 24-hour supervision of individuals who, because of old age or impairments, necessarily need assistance with the activities of daily living.

Respite

The in-home care of a chronically ill beneficiary intended to give the caregiver a rest. Can also be provided by a hospice or a nursing facility.

Respite Care

Includes any temporary service which lets caregivers take a break from caring for people with disabilities, illnesses, dementia or other health problems while a third party assumes the regular caregiver's role. Types of respite include having someone come into the home so that the caregiver can relax or run errands; providing out-of-home respite through adult day programs for the impaired relative; and/or extending overnight respite opportunities (in-home or out-of-home) so that the caregiver can extend relief.

S

Senior Care Manager

Also known as case managers or geriatric care managers, these professionals (social workers, nurses, gerontologists or other professionals trained to work as care managers with older adults) provide on-going services such as coordinating all aspects of the elder's care with the client, family, doctor and service providers. Services also includes in-home assessments, written plans of care, and initiating and regular monitoring of services being provided to the elder. Some care management agencies provide additional services such as transportation or 24 hour on-call nursing care. They may offer conservatorship and/or guardianship when requested and decreed necessary by a District Court. Payment may come from private, special project, grant or governmental funds

Skilled Care

Institutional care (a subset of post-acute care) that is less intensive than hospital care in its nursing and medical service, but which includes procedures whose administration requires the training and skills of an RN. This care is usually needed 24 hours a day, must be ordered by a physician, and must follow a plan of care. Individuals usually get skilled care in a nursing home but may also receive it in other places. "Higher level" of care (such as injections, catheterizations, and dressing changes) provided by trained medical professionals, including nurses, doctors, and physical therapist. Both Medicare and Medicaid reimburse for care at the skilled level. Medicare reimburses 100 days of skilled care following an acute hospitalization. This is commonly available in designated beds in a nursing home.

Skilled Nursing Care

Skilled care that is administered or supervised by Registered Nurses. Skilled nursing care can include: intravenous injections, tube feeding, and changing sterile dressings on a wound. Any service that could be safely done by an average non-medical person without the supervision of a Registered Nurse is not considered skilled care.

Skilled Nursing Facility

Also known as nursing homes, convalescent hospitals and/or rest homes, SNFs provide continuous (24-hour) nursing services (care and rehabilitation in addition to regular medical services) under a registered nurse or licensed vocational nurse. They are equipped to provide more extensive care needs, such as administering injections, monitoring blood pressure, and caring for patients on ventilators, or those requiring intravenous feeding. However, many residents in skilled nursing facilities may be receiving only "custodial" care such as help with bathing, eating, getting in and out of bed, and using the toilet. In addition, SNFs must provide recreational activities for residents. They may also provide rehabilitative services, such as physical, occupational, or speech therapies. SNF care can be costly (an average of $40,000 per year).

Social Health Maintenance Organization

Known as SHMO, this organization provides a unique alternative to traditional HMO by combining preventive, acute and long-term care benefits. A managed system of health and long-term care services geared toward an elderly client population. Under this model, a single provider entity assumes responsibility for a full range of acute inpatient, ambulatory, rehabilitative, extended home health and personal care services under a fixed budget, which is determined prospectively. Elderly people who reside in the target service area are voluntarily enrolled. Once enrolled, individuals are obligated to receive all SHMO covered services through SHMO providers, similar to the operation of a medical model health maintenance organization.

Social Security Disability Insurance

A system (known as SSDI) of federally provided payments to eligible workers (and, in some cases, their families) when they are unable to continue working because of a disability. Benefits begin with the sixth full month of disability and continue until the individual is capable of substantial gainful activity.

Special Care Units

Designated area of a residential care facility or nursing home that cares specifically for the needs of people with Alzheimer's, head injuries, dementia, or other specific disorders.

Spend Down

Under the Medicaid program, a method by which an individual establishes Medicaid eligibility by reducing gross income through incurring medical expenses until net income (after medical expenses) meets Medicaid financial requirements. A resident spends down when he/she is no longer sufficiently covered by a third-party payer (usually Medicare) and has exhausted all personal assets. The resident then becomes eligible for Medicaid coverage.

Subacute Care

Serves patients needing complex care or rehabilitation. Subacute care (also known as transitional care) is defined as comprehensive inpatient care designed for someone who has an acute illness, injury or exacerbation of a disease process. It is goal oriented treatment rendered immediately after, or instead of, acute hospitalization to treat one or more specific active complex medical conditions or to administer one or more technically complex treatments, in the context of a person's underlying long-term conditions and overall situation. Subacute care may include long-term ventilator care or other procedures provided on a routine basis either at home or by trained staff at a skilled nursing facility. Subacute care is generally more intensive than traditional nursing facility care and less than acute care. It requires frequent (daily to weekly) recurrent patient assessment and review of the clinical course and treatment plan for a limited (several days to several months) time period until the condition is stabilized or a predetermined treatment course is completed.

Supplemental Security Income

Known as SSI, this program may provide monthly disability income for those who meet Social Security rules for disability who have limited income and resources. A public assistance program providing support for low-income aged, blind and disabled persons, established by Title XVI of the Social Security Act. SSI replaced state welfare programs for the aged, blind and disabled in since 1972, with a federally administered program, paying a monthly basic benefit nationwide of $284.30 for an individual and $426.40 for a couple in 1983. States may supplement this basic benefit amount.

T

Term Life Insurance

Provides coverage for individuals for a period of one or more years. Pays a death benefit only if individual dies during that term. It does not typically build cash value.

Third Party Notice

A policy provision that allows the policyholder name someone who the insurance company would notify if coverage were about to end because premiums haven't been paid. This individual can be a relative, friend, or professional such as a lawyer or accountant.

Title III Services

Services provided to individuals 60 years of age and older which are funded under Title III of the Older Americans Act. Include: congregate and home-delivered meals, supportive services (e.g., transportation, information and referral, legal assistance, and more), in-home services (e.g., homemaker services, personal care, chore services, and more), and health promotion/disease prevention services (e.g., health screenings, exercise programs, and more).

Title XIX

Part of Medicaid, this is a federal and state-funded program of medical assistance to low-income individuals of all ages. There are income eligibility requirements for Medicaid.

Title XVIII

Part of Medicare, this is a federal health insurance program for persons age 65 and over (and certain disabled persons under age 65). Consists of 2 parts: Part A (hospital insurance) and Part B (optional medical insurance which covers physicians' services and outpatient care in part and which requires beneficiaries to pay a monthly premium).

Title XX Services

Known as Social Services Block Grant services. Grants given to states under the Social Security Act which fund limited amounts of social services for people of all ages (including some in-home services, abuse prevention services, and more). States are given wide discretion to determine the services to be provided and the groups that may be eligible for services, usually low income families and individuals.

Transfer of Assets

Transfer of a potential Medicaid recipient's money or possessions to a third party, which may be interpreted under state and federal Medicaid law as an attempt to qualify the person for Medicaid when he/she would not otherwise be eligible. Medicaid regulations govern time frames and conditions which individuals may transfer assets to others without jeopardizing Medicaid eligibility.

Transitional Care

Transitional care can be defined as that which is required to facilitate a shift from one disease stage and/or place of care to another. Also known as post-acute care or subacute care, a type of short-term care provided by many long-term care facilities and hospitals which may include rehabilitation services, specialized care for certain diseases, conditions and/or post-surgical care and other services associated with the transition between the hospital and home. Residents on these units often have been hospitalized recently and typically have more complicated medical needs. The goal of subacute care is to discharge residents to their homes or to a lower level of care.

Trust

A legal title to property held by one party for the benefit of another. An arrangement in which an individual (the trustor) gives fiduciary control of property to a person or institution (the trustee) for the benefit of one or more beneficiaries. The property so held is known as a trust.

Trustee

An individual, organization or institution (such as a bank or law firm) designated in a trust document to administer and/or manage the assets held in the trust for the benefit of the trust's beneficiary or beneficiaries.

Trustor

And individual, organization or institution (such as a bank), that holds legal title to property in order to administer it for a beneficiary

TTY

A text telephone system that allows a hearing-impaired user to type messages (data), one character at a time, to another person and read responses on a small screen. Similar to cell phone text messaging, a "read only" conversation can exist between two people who each use the equipment. An option is having a non-hearing-impaired caller utilize This term refers to a means of sending data one character at a time. a relay service where a special operator acts as a go-between to translate the speaker's words into text and text print into voice communication.

U

Universal Life Insurance

Flexible type of policy that allows individuals to periodically adjust their premium payments and the amount of coverage.

V

Veterans Benefit Information Online

Military Records Request

http://www.archives.gov

National Cemetery Administration

http://www.cem.va.gov/

VA Facility Directory

http://www1.va.gov

Veterans Health Administration

http://www.appc1.va.gov

Veterans Benefits Administration

http://www.va.gov/

Federal Benefits For Veterans

http://www1.va.gov/opa/vadocs/Fed-ben.pdf

Visiting Nurse Association

A voluntary health agency that is a not-for-profit organization providing intermittent, skilled care in the home under orders from your physician.

Basic services include health supervision, education and counseling; beside care; and the carrying out of physicians orders. Personnel include nurses and home health aides who are trained for specific tasks of personal bedside care. These agencies are committed to providing the finest home health care available, regardless of an individual's ability to pay.

W

Whole Life Insurance

Policies that build cash value and cover a person for as long as he or she lives if premiums continue to be paid.

LIVING WILL DECLARATION (SAMPLE*)

THIS DECLARATION is made by ___________________________

(Typed or printed notary name)

As I make this declaration I am of sound mind.

I direct this declaration to my family and to anyone else who may become responsible for my health, welfare, financial, or other affairs. I hereby declare as follows:

- Should circumstances come to exist such that there is no reasonable expectation of my recovery, I direct that no extreme measures of kind be used.
- In the event that there is a substantial question about the possibility of my recovery, or if there is no reasonable expectation of my recovery, I request that medication or other measures be utilized to reduce my physical suffering.
- I ask that this request be carried out even in the event that such measures or such medication may shorten my life.
- On behalf of my estate and myself, I hereby release from any liability all hospitals, physicians, other medical personnel, and all other individuals having any part in complying with the requests made hereinabove.

It is my intention that this declaration shall be valid until revoked by me.

SIGNED this ____ day of ____________, 20____.

(signature)____

(typed legal name)__________________________________

Residing at:_______________________________________

This Declarant is known to me and voluntarily signed this document in my presence.

WITNESS:____

Residing at: _______________________________________

WITNESS:____

Residing at: _______________________________________

STATE OF ________________) COUNTY OF ______________)

SUBSCRIBED, SWORN TO AND ACKNOWLEDGED before me by ____________, the Declarant, and subscribed and sworn to before me by the above-named witnesses, this _____ day of _______________, 20_____ .

____

(Notary signature)

____

(Typed or printed notary name)

(SEAL) Notary Public for the State of ________________

Residing at: _____________________________________

My commission expires: ______________________ (date)

***NOTE:** DC Press does not offer legal advice. Prior to attempting to utilize any form presented in this book or when making an important decision effecting your future healthcare or finances, seek the advise of a legal, accounting, and/or medical professionals.

DURABLE HEALTH CARE POWER OF ATTORNEY AND HEALTH CARE TREATMENT INSTRUCTIONS LIVING WILL*

NOTE: On Making Healthcare Decisions:

You have the right to decide the type of healthcare you want. Should you become unable to make, understand, or communicate decisions about medical care, your wishes for medical treatment are most likely to be followed if you have expressed those wishes in writing in advance by:

(1) Naming a health care agent to decide treatment for you; and

(2) Giving health care treatment instructions to your health care agent or health care provider.

An advance healthcare directive is a written set of instructions that express your wishes for medical treatment. It may contain a

> ***NOTE:** DC Press does not offer legal advice. Prior to attempting to utilize any form presented in this book or when making an important decision effecting your future healthcare or finances, seek the advise of a legal, accounting, and/or medical professionals.

healthcare power of attorney, where you name a person called a healthcare agent to decide treatment for you, and a living will, where you tell your *healthcare agent* and healthcare providers your choices regarding the initiation, continuation, withholding, or withdrawal of treatment that would sustain life and other specific instructions.

You may limit your healthcare agent's involvement in deciding your medical treatment so that your healthcare agent will speak for you only when you are unable to speak for yourself or you may give your healthcare agent the power to speak for you immediately.

NOTE: The form that follows below is a combination of a durable power of attorney and a living will. It permits your healthcare agent the power to speak on your behalf, when you are unable to do so for yourself.

A living will cannot be followed unless your attending physician determines that you lack the ability to understand, make, and communicate health care decisions for yourself and you are either permanently unconscious or you have an end-stage medical condition (a condition that will result in death despite the introduction or continuation of medical treatment).

You, and not your healthcare agent, remain responsible for the cost of your medical care. If you do not write down your wishes about your healthcare in advance, and if later you become unable to understand, make, or communicate these decisions, those wishes may not be honored because they may remain unknown to others.

A health care provider who refuses to honor your wishes about healthcare must tell you of its refusal and help to transfer you to a health care provider who will honor your wishes.

You should give a copy of your advance health care directive — a living will, healthcare power of attorney or a document containing both — to your healthcare agent, your physicians, family members, and others you expect would likely attend to your needs if you become unable to understand, make, or communicate decisions about medical care.

If your health care wishes change, tell your physician and write a new advance healthcare directive to replace your old one. It is important in selecting a healthcare agent that you choose a person you trust who is likely to be available in a medical situation where you cannot make decisions for yourself. You should inform that person that you have appointed him or her as your healthcare agent and discuss your beliefs and values with him or her so that your healthcare agent will understand your health care objectives.

You may wish to consult with knowledgeable, trusted individuals such as family members, your physician and/or clergy when considering an expression of your values and health care wishes. You are free to create your own advance health care directive to convey your wishes regarding medical treatment.

NOTE: This form is an example of an advance health care directive that combines a living will with a healthcare power of attorney.

Using this form:

If you decide to use this form or create your own advance healthcare directive, you should consult with your physician and your attorney to make sure that your wishes are clearly expressed and comply with the law.

If you decide to use this form but disagree with any of its statements, you may cross out those statements. You may add comments to this form or use your own form to help your physician or healthcare agent decide your medical care.

This form is designed to give your health care agent broad powers to make health care decisions for you whenever you cannot make them for yourself. It is also designed to express a desire to limit or authorize care if you have an end-stage medical condition or are permanently unconscious.

If you do not desire to give your healthcare agent broad powers, or you do not wish to limit your care if you have an end-stage medical condition or are permanently unconscious, you may wish to use a different form or create your own. You should also use a different form if you wish to express your preferences in more detail than this form allows or if you wish for your healthcare agent to be able to speak for you immediately. In these situations, it is particularly important that you consult with your attorney and physician to make sure that your wishes are clearly expressed.

This form allows you to tell your healthcare agent your goals if you have an end-stage medical condition or other extreme and irreversible medical condition, such as advanced cancer or Alzheimer's disease. Do you want medical care applied aggressively in these situations or would you consider such aggressive medical care burdensome and undesirable?

You may choose whether you want your health care agent to be bound by your instructions or whether you want your healthcare agent to be able to decide at the time what course of treatment the healthcare agent thinks most fully reflects your wishes and values.

If you are a woman and are pregnant at the time a healthcare decision would otherwise be made pursuant to this form, you need to ask about the laws of your state or commonwealth that might prohibit implementation of that decision if it directs that life-sustaining treatment, including nutrition and hydration, be withheld or withdrawn from you, unless your attending physician and an obstetrician who have examined you certify in your medical record that the life-sustaining treatment:

(1) Will not maintain you in such a way as to permit the continuing development and live birth of the unborn child;

(2) Will be physically harmful to you; or

(3) Will cause pain to you that cannot be alleviated by medication.

Nevertheless, investigate the specific laws that apply in your state or commonwealth where you reside.

DURABLE HEALTH CARE POWER OF ATTORNEY (SAMPLE)*

I,________________________________, of________________County, ________________State, appoint the person named below to be my healthcare agent to make health and personal care decisions for me.

Effective immediately and continuously until my death or revocation by a writing signed by me or someone authorized to make healthcare treatment decisions for me, I authorize all healthcare providers or other covered entities to disclose to my health care agent, upon my agent's request, any information, oral or written, regarding my physical or mental health, including, but not limited to, medical and hospital records and what is otherwise private, privileged, protected or personal health information, such as health information as defined and described in the Health Insurance Portability and Accountability Act of 1996 (Public Law 104-191, 110 Stat. 1936), the regulations promulgated thereunder and any other State or local laws and rules. Information disclosed by a healthcare

***NOTE:** DC Press does not offer legal advice. Prior to attempting to utilize any form presented in this book or when making an important decision effecting your future healthcare or finances, seek the advise of a legal, accounting, and/or medical professionals.

provider or other covered entity may be re-disclosed and may no longer be subject to the privacy rules provided by 45 C.F.R. Pt. 164.

The remainder of this document will take effect when and only when I lack the ability to understand, make or communicate a choice regarding a health or personal care decision as verified by my attending physician. My healthcare agent may not delegate the authority to make decisions.

MY HEALTHCARE AGENT HAS ALL OF THE FOLLOWING POWERS SUBJECT TO THE HEALTH CARE TREATMENT INSTRUCTIONS THAT FOLLOW.

(**NOTE:** Cross out or remove any powers you do not want to give your healthcare agent):

1. To authorize, withhold or withdraw medical care and surgical procedures.
2. To authorize, withhold or withdraw nutrition (food) or hydration (water) medically supplied by tube through my nose, stomach, intestines, arteries or veins.
3. To authorize my admission to or discharge from a medical, nursing, residential or similar facility and to make agreements for my care and health insurance for my care, including hospice and/or palliative care.
4. To hire and fire medical, social service and other support personnel responsible for my care.
5. To take any legal action necessary to do what I have directed.
6. To request that a physician responsible for my care issue a do-not-resuscitate (DNR) order, including an out-of-hospital DNR order, and sign any required documents and consents.

APPOINTMENT OF HEALTH CARE AGENT (SAMPLE*)

I appoint the following healthcare agent:

____

(Name and relationship)

Address:_______________________________________

Telephone Number: ______________________________

Home:____

Work: ____

E-MAIL:_______________________________________

NOTE: If you do not name a healthcare agent, healthcare providers will ask your family or an adult who knows your preferences and life values for help in determining (interpreting) your wishes for treatment.

> ***NOTE:** DC Press does not offer legal advice. Prior to attempting to utilize any form presented in this book or when making an important decision effecting your future healthcare or finances, seek the advise of a legal, accounting, and/or medical professionals.

NOTE: You may not appoint your doctor or other healthcare provider as your healthcare agent, unless they are related to you by blood, marriage or adoption.

If my healthcare agent is not readily available or if my healthcare agent is my spouse and an action for divorce is filed by either of us after the date of this document, I appoint the person or persons named below in the order named. (NOTE: It can be helpful, but not required, to name alternative healthcare agents.)

First Alternative HealthCare Agent:

____

(Name and relationship)

Address:______________________________________

Telephone Number: _____________________________

Home:____

Work: ____

E-MAIL:______________________________________

Second Alternative HealthCare Agent:

____

(Name and relationship)

Address:______________________________________

Telephone Number: _____________________________

Home:____

Work: ____

E-MAIL:______________________________________

CONCLUSION

To the Reader:

Always remember this quotation:

The opposite of Love is not Hate — but Indifference.

People filling out this book — in order to help make their loved ones' lives a little easier — are certainly not "Indifferent."

This book is meant to be a "Hands-on-Tool" to be utilized during your lifetime, a reference for your decedants, and a guide for your future caregivers.

The time you take now to complete this book will be appreciated by so many in the future.

Good Luck!

Dee Marrella

PART VIII

Notes

The following space is provided for individuals to add all of the "extra information" that hasn't been presented in other parts of this guide – or to embellish things said earlier but requiring additional space. Anything goes here. Feel free to give future caregivers more insight into the real you.

NOTES

NOTES

NOTES

NOTES

NOTES

NOTES

NOTES

NOTES

NOTES

NOTES

NOTES

ABOUT THE AUTHOR

Dee Marrella has experienced life as a military wife and a corporate wife and as a result has seen much of the world and experienced many varied cultures. Born in Paterson, New Jersey, Dee spent twenty plus years in the field of education in both Europe and the United States. Experiencing these different cultures afforded her the opportunity to observe vast differences in the ways caregivers interact with both young and old individuals within societies.

In 1994 it was medically necessary for Dee's mother to enter a nursing home. Dee's constant presence at the home, watching so many caregivers deal with pain, love and guilt gave her the inspiration to create ***Who Cares.*** After two editions, ***Who Cares*** is now in its third edition and newly entitled, ***The Me You Don't Know***.

Dee resides in Wyomissing, PA with her husband Len. They are proud parents of three grown daughters who have given them seven grandchildren.

If you found this book thought provoking and there is an interest in having the author speak to your organization, please feel free to contact her at:

Dee Marrella
Contact Information
(610) 478-3000
(610) 288-5801 (fax)
dee@themeyoudontknow.com
www.themeyoudontknow.com

www.FocusOnEthics.com